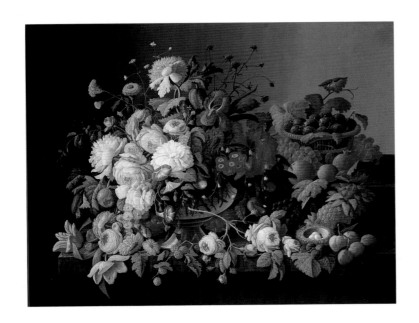

Scents of Time

PERFUME
from Ancient Egypt to the 21st Century

Edwin T. Morris

THE METROPOLITAN MUSEUM OF ART
Bulfinch Press/Little, Brown and Company
Boston • New York • London

The works of art reproduced in this book are from the collections of The Metropolitan Museum of Art unless otherwise noted.

COVER DETAIL AND TITLE PAGE: *Still Life: Flowers and Fruit*
Severin Roesen, German, active in America 1848–1872
Oil on canvas, 40 x 50⅜ in., 1850–55
Purchase, Bequest of Charles Allen Munn, by exchange, Fosburgh Fund Inc. and
Mr. and Mrs. J. William Middendorf II Gifts, and Henry G. Keasbey Bequest, 1967   67.111

TABLE OF CONTENTS: *Lotus* (detail)
Zhang Daqian, Chinese, 1899–1983
Hanging scroll, ink and color on paper, 59½ x 28 1/16 in., 1946
Gift of Robert Hatfield Ellsworth, in memory of La Ferne Hatfield Ellsworth, 1986   1986.267.360

ঌ

Published by The Metropolitan Museum of Art and Bulfinch Press
Bulfinch Press is an imprint and trademark of Little, Brown and Company (Inc.)

ISBN 0-87099-898-6 (MMA)
ISBN 0-8212-2635-5 (Bulfinch Press)

Library of Congress Catalog Card Number 99-73036

Produced by the Department of Special Publications, The Metropolitan Museum of Art.
Robie Rogge, Publishing Manager; Judith Cressy, Editor; Anna Raff, Designer;
Lauren Wolfe, Editorial Assistant; Alix MacGowan, Production Associate.
All photography by The Metropolitan Museum of Art Photograph Studio unless otherwise noted.

Historic scents created for The Metropolitan Museum of Art by Givaudan Roure Fragrances

Scents of Time is packaged with eight bottled fragrances. Ingredients: SD alcohol 40B
(alcohol denat.), fragrance, water. Attention: flammable. Do not take internally. Keep
out of the reach of children. Product may cause allergic reaction in some people.

Visit the Museum's web site: www.metmuseum.org
Visit the Bulfinch Press web site: www.bulfinchpress.com

First Edition
Printed in Hong Kong
10 9 8 7 6 5 4 3 2

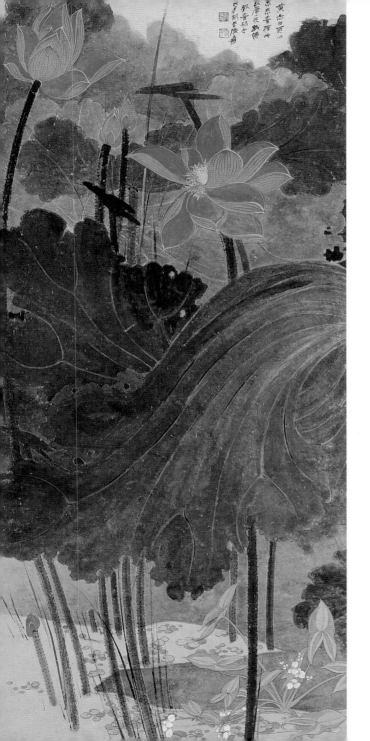

Table of Contents

Introduction   5

Scent in the Fertile Crescent   15

Scent in the Classical World   27

Scent in the East   39

Scent in East Asia   51

Scent in the Middle Ages and the Renaissance   61

Scent in the Eighteenth Century   73

Scent in the Nineteenth Century   83

Scent in the Belle Époque and the Jazz Age   91

Scent from the Thirties to the Present   103

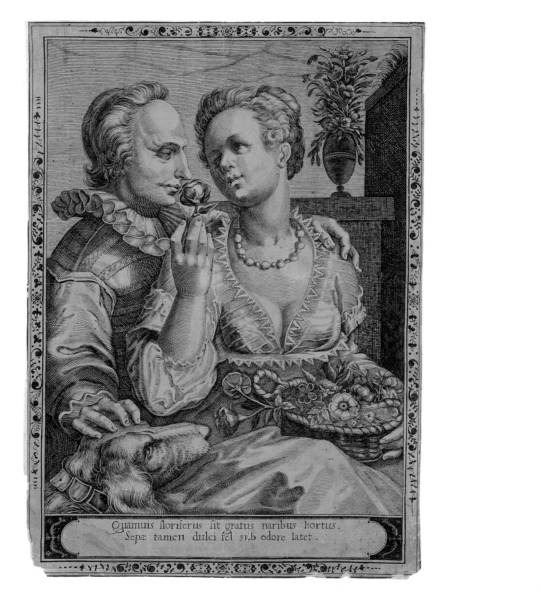

Quamuis floriferus sit gratus naribus hortus,
Sepæ tamen dulci fel sub odore latet.

Comme d'autres esprits voguent sur la musique,
Le mien, ô mon amour! nage sur ton parfum.

As the spirits of certain people hover over music,
My soul, o my love! swims on your perfume.

Charles Baudelaire, "La Chevelure"

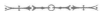

Perfume has been with us for more than four thousand years—lingering in unexpected places, evoking memory and desire. Its story draws from cultures the world over: The art of blending scents originated in the ancient Near East, traveled west to Greece and Rome, and was dependent on the Arabian trade in aromatics that penetrated to East Asia. The first center of European perfumery was Renaissance Italy, but France took precedence in the eighteenth century. Today the United States shares the spotlight with France as an important producer of fragrance.

The rose has been the flower of romance and the favorite scent in perfumery from ancient times to the present. This 16th-century engraving, *The Sense of Smell*, was made by an anonymous artist, as a reverse copy of an engraving by Jan Saenredam after Hendrick Goltzius.
Purchase, Harry G. Friedman Bequest, 1967 67.539.391

In all cultures and periods, craftspeople have lavished their skills creating containers for perfume. Beautiful bottles and jars have always been made to reflect perfume's costliness and rarity. Vials and other perfume containers, made of glass, clay, stone, and precious metals, have been carefully preserved for millennia—some have even accompanied their owners to the tomb. Collectively, the accoutrements of perfume reflect in miniature all the arts, vanities, and changing styles of civilization.

There is a wonderful continuity to the story of fragrance, for while the technical aspects of gathering and blending scent have developed considerably over the centuries, in many other ways perfumery has changed very little. The scents that Cleopatra enjoyed are still enjoyed today. Jasmine flowers continue to be culled by hand, roses are still pampered and picked at dawn, and as always, patchouli is cured long enough to bring forth its characteristic earthy scent. The very materials that were once held in the bottles and flasks of antiquity, shown on the pages of this book, are still part of modern perfumery.

THE EIGHT FRAGRANCES OF *Scents of Time*

The fragrances included with this book have been specially blended to capture the essences of eight of the most influential scents in history.

Frankincense is a resin from southern Arabia with a warm, balsamic scent. The resin was used as an incense by Queen Hatshepsut, Alexander the Great, and the Roman Caesars. It was carried to China and later to Renaissance Italy, where its fragrance as incense was admired. Today, frankincense is often an ingredient in oriental-type perfumes.

Rose is called the queen of fragrances and is one of the most widely enjoyed essences in the world. The ancient Greeks, Romans, and Persians were enthusiastic about perfumes made from the flower. Rose water was used for rinsing the hands in Renaissance Italy and in Elizabethan England. The scent of rose was a particular favorite of Queen Elizabeth I.

Sandalwood-Jasmine represents the enormous botanical contribution of India and Kashmir to perfumery.

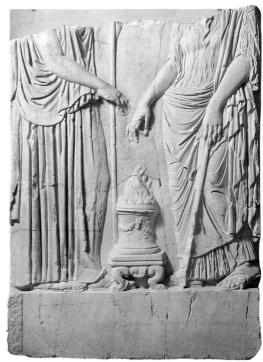

The aroma of burning incense was enjoyed throughout the classical world and was part of every important ceremony. This marble relief fragment is a Roman adaptation (ca. 1st–2nd centuries A.D.) of a Greek relief (ca. 350–325 B.C.) showing the major deities of the sanctuary at Eleusis.
Fletcher Fund, 1924 24.97.99

Sandalwood's sensual, warm odor has appeared in perfume for two thousand years. Jasmine's heady, full-bodied floral quality is associated with the rise of perfumery in the Renaissance and has made an appearance in many of the *grands parfums* of the twentieth century.

香 **Orange Blossom** originated in East Asia and was later introduced into the Mediterranean region. The light, floral scent of orange blossom is a key ingredient in eau de cologne. Neroli, the oil distilled from the orange blossom, was the scent of choice for the perfumed leather gloves of the Middle Ages and the Renaissance.

♖ **Spice** is made up of aromatics gathered from the Near East and the Far East. In the fifteenth century, Europeans spared no effort in importing cloves, cinnamon, nutmeg, and ginger. The spices were mixed into potpourris to add scent to a room or were carried on the person in pomanders. Oriental-type compositions are among the twentieth-century perfumes with a rich spice note.

⚜ **Eau de Cologne** is the longest-lived perfumery creation on the market today. All true eaux de cologne derive from the formula brought out by the Farina family in 1709. The composition was a particular favorite of Madame du Barry and, later, Napoléon. Eau de cologne's clean, sparkling tones remain enormously popular.

🌹 **Millefleurs** blended with aldehydes represents modern perfumery. The development of the solvent extraction process in the late nineteenth century enabled perfumers to draw on many new floral essences; millefleurs compositions, or floral bouquets, reflect this broad range of flowers. In the 1920s, aldehydes, synthetics that have a bright, effervescent note, were added to the medley, complementing the floral quality.

● **Sportif** reflects today's growing interest in fitness. This trend has led to the introduction of many perfume blends with a clean, fresh note. Oils from the zests of citrus fruits frequently appear in the new sportif compositions.

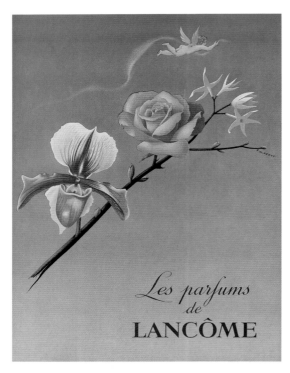

Fine perfumes are composed of many scents, as suggested by the advertisement above. Sometimes several hundred botanical oils and synthetics are blended to create a single perfume. Blending ensures that a perfume will develop and change as it remains on the skin over time. The scent of the top note appears first, the middle note minutes later, and the base note later still.

From *Femina*, March–April 1952. The Metropolitan Museum of Art, Irene Lewisohn Costume Reference Library

WHAT IS PERFUME?

Until the technique for distilling alcohol was perfected in Italy in about 1320, perfumes were produced with an oil or animal fat base and were used as lotions and pomades for the body and hair. Today, "perfume" is defined as a mixture of twenty-two to thirty percent essential oil in ethyl alcohol, with a slight amount of water. An eau de toilette contains five to fifteen percent essential oil in ethyl alcohol and water, and an eau de cologne has less than five percent essential oil in the alcohol-water mix. Compared to other varieties of scent, true perfumes are longer-lasting on the skin and are more expensive because they contain a greater percentage of essential oils.

FRAGRANCE FAMILIES

The dominant impression created by a perfume determines which fragrance family it belongs to. The families and some of the perfumes that represent them are described below.

Aldehydic: Aldehydic or "modern" perfumes are those with the arresting scent of aldehydes, synthetic compounds with clean, diffusive, sparkling notes. Aldehydes are usually associated with florals and women's perfumes. Perfumes of this type include Chanel No. 5, L'Interdit, Arpège, Rive Gauche, White Linen, and Cerruti Femme 1881.

Chypre: "Chypre" is the French name for the island of Cyprus, the legendary birthplace of Venus. Chypre-type perfumes are sophisticated, earthy, classic scents that are based on an accord, several scents that blend together so perfectly they are treated as a single scent. The two scents that are included in all accords are patchouli and oakmoss. A classic chypre-type perfume might be blended of bergamot, oakmoss, sandalwood, patchouli, and labdanum, and floralized with jasmine and rose. Women's chypre-type perfumes include Miss Dior, Femme, Cabochard, and Ysatis. Men's colognes of this type include Polo and Montana.

Citrus: This family of perfumes comprises the familiar fresh, crisp scent of bergamot, as well as that of lemon, orange, tangerine, and grapefruit peels. Citrus is particularly recognizable in many men's fragrances, including Monsieur de Givenchy, Armani, and Eau Sauvage. Women's citrus scents include Dior's Eau Fraîche, Eau de Patou and Ô de Lancôme. Many citrus scents, such as 4711, are unisex in character.

Floral: This category, the most popular in perfumery, includes both single floral scents and floral bouquets, which weave scents together. Floral scents, led by rose, jasmine, and tuberose, can be rich in character or light and airy. They predominate in women's perfumes such as Joy, L'Air du Temps, Fracas, Fidji, Giorgio, and Blonde.

Fougère: *Fougère* means "fern" in French. This family is characterized by bracing, herbaceous scents that appear mainly in men's colognes. Paco Rabanne, Cool Water, and Michael Jordan belong to this family.

Fruity Floral: This is one of the new perfume families, a modern outgrowth of the floral group used mainly in women's fragrances. Fruity

A PERFUME TIME LINE

1800 B.C. The maceration process is used to make perfume in Mesopotamia.

1400 B.C. Glassmaking is discovered in western Asia.

356–323 B.C. Alexander the Great introduces plants of the Persian empire into Europe. Theophrastus of Athens writes the first book on scent.

A.D. 1–100 Romans perfect the art of blown glass.

200–300 Alchemists in Alexandria develop the first still.

980–1037 The Muslim Ibn-Sina perfects the distillation process used to extract oil of rose.

1320 Italian distillers invent the serpentine cooler, which allows for the commercial production of alcohol of high proof.

1370 Hungary Water, the first named alcohol-based perfume, is produced.

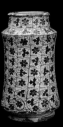

1533 Caterina de' Medici brings the art of perfumery from Italy to France when she marries King Henri II.

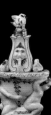

1709 The Farina family creates eau de cologne.

European techniques for making porcelain are perfected in Meissen, Germany.

1715–74 Louis XV's "perfumed court" stimulates the commercial cultivation of flowers for perfumery in the south of France.

1835 Solvent extraction of scent is perfected.

1868 The first synthetic scents are developed.

1910 Paul Poiret forges the link between couture and fragrance.

1921 Chanel No. 5 is the first perfume containing aldehydes.

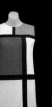

1960–80 The "designer revolution" links mass marketing and couture.

1980–present Designers launch "lifestyle" fragrances. Aromatherapy gains widespread popularity.

florals are youthful, blending floral notes with fresh fruity notes like peach. They are represented by Lauren and Amazone, among others.

Green: "Green" fragrances are characterized by a fresh, natural, "outdoors" scent and can include pine, mint, and herbal notes. Green women's perfumes include Vent Vert, Chanel No. 19, Alfred Sung, and Safari. Grey Flannel and Fahrenheit are men's fragrances with green notes.

Leather/Chypre: The distinct scent of leather combined with chypre-type accords appears in a number of sophisticated, classic perfumes. Perfumers create the scent of leather with oil of birch tar and synthetics. Women's perfumes of this type include Bandit, Miss Dior, Équipage, and Calèche. Aramis is a leather/chypre men's cologne.

Musk: The musk family is characterized by its sensual, warm, clean notes. At one time musk oil came from the glands of the musk deer; today the scent is re-created synthetically. Gendarme is a men's cologne with musk notes. Jovan's Musk and CK Be are unisex colognes of this family.

Oriental: The oriental family represents warm, spicy, long-lasting women's perfumes with several subgroups. Amber orientals have notes of vanilla and "amber," synthetic ambergris. (True ambergris, which comes from whales, has not been used in perfumery for more than thirty years.) Amber orientals include Shalimar, Must de Cartier, and Obsession. Spicy orientals are rich with clove, nutmeg, and cinnamon, and include Shocking, Youth Dew, and Opium. Florientals, as the name suggests, combine two favorite fragrance families. L'Heure Bleue, Oscar, Bijan, Lou Lou, and Nicole Miller are all part of this subgroup. Sheer florientals, the most recently developed subgroup, are lighter in scent than other oriental-type perfumes, though just as long lasting on the skin. One member of the sheer-floriental subgroup is Allure.

TECHNIQUES

Since ancient times, perfumers have used a variety of means to utilize essential oils from plants and other natural materials.

Distillation is key to fragrance production. For this process, flowers and other plant parts are put into a still and boiled with water or subjected to steam. The plant parts' essential oils turn to gas and rise with the water vapors to the top of the still. When the gas and vapors cool, they turn to liquid and collect in the condenser. The oil and water separate and can then be decanted. Many delicate flowers cannot withstand the heat of distillation.

Enfleurage was known and practiced in ancient Egypt. In the eighteenth and nineteenth centuries, it was vital to the development of the perfumery industry in Grasse, France. Performed at room temperature, enfleurage is effective in extracting delicate floral oils that heat and distillation would harm. In this process, purified fat, such as a blend of lard and tallow, is spread on a glass plate, then flowers are placed on the fat, which absorbs the floral scent. Several times over the course of twenty-four hours, the flowers are replaced with fresh ones. When the fat has become saturated with floral scent, it is washed with alcohol; then the fat is chilled and the scent is removed with the alcohol by filtering. Enfleurage remained in use until the early twentieth century, when it was largely replaced by solvent extraction (see below).

1990–present Headspace technology emerges. The United States begins to rival France in fragrance creation.

Page 9 top:
Cast-bronze cosmetic container made in the area of southeastern Iran or Afghanistan in the 2nd millennium B.C.
Gift of Sheldon Lewis Breithart, 1983
1983.535.36 A

Page 9 center:
Roman blown-glass *alabastron*, or perfume bottle, made from fused glass rods.
Gift of J. Pierpont Morgan, 1917   17.194.286

Page 9 bottom:
Apothecary jar (*albarello*). Made in Valencia, Spain, in the 15th century.
The Cloisters Collection, 1956   56.171.91
Photograph by Schecter Lee

Page 10 top:
Scent bottle in the shape of a fountain. Made at the Chelsea factory, England, in the mid-18th century.
Gift of Irwin Untermyer, 1971   1971.75.22

Page 10 center:
The scent of lilacs and several other flowers can appear in perfumery only through synthetics.
Lilacs in a Window (Vase de Lilas à la Fenêtre), ca. 1880–83; Mary Cassatt, American, 1884–1926.
Partial and Promised Gift of Susan and Douglas Dillon, 1997   1997.207

Page 10 bottom:
"Mondrian" day dress by Yves Saint Laurent, fall 1965; red, blue, white, yellow, and black wool jersey. Saint Laurent is the designer behind Opium, Rive Gauche, and many other perfumes.
Gift of Mrs. William Rand, 1969   CI.69.23

Expression is the most common technique for extracting essential oils from the peels of citrus fruits. The peels are cold pressed under a spray of water and then filtered for use. The heat required in distillation would damage the intensity of most citrus-peel oils.

Headspace technology is a gas chromatographic technique perfected in the 1970s, whereby a living plant is encapsulated—on-site or in a laboratory—and its fragrance chemically analyzed. Thus, without destroying a plant or changing its character, perfumers can determine the composition of a plant's scent at its peak and reproduce it synthetically.

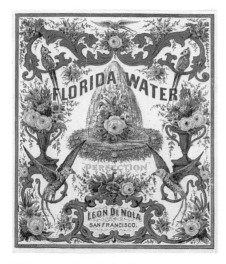

When the first alcohol-based perfumes were made in Italy in the 14th century, they were called waters because of alcohol's resemblance to water. The name has remained associated with perfumery, as this 19th-century American label makes clear.

The Jefferson R. Burdick Collection, Gift of Jefferson R. Burdick   Album 34

Maceration is similar to enfleurage (see above) but is performed at higher temperatures. In this process, flowers and other plant parts are warmed in hot vegetable oils or animal fats. The mixture is then filtered and allowed to cool. Before the development of alcohol-based perfumes, maceration was the principal means of creating perfumed oils for the skin and hair.

Solvent extraction was developed in the 1830s as a means of removing essential oils from flowers that cannot withstand the heat of distillation. Flowers are placed in a sealed tank into which petroleum ether is pumped. The ether acts as a "dry cleaner," dissolving the essential oils and odorless plant paraffins, or waxes on a flower's surface. When the ether is evaporated out of the tank, what remains is a floral "concrete"—essential oils solidified in wax. To separate the essential oils from the wax, the concrete is washed in alcohol and chilled, the wax hardens, and the scented alcohol is filtered off. Next, the alcohol is evaporated under a vacuum, leaving behind an absolute, or highly concentrated floral essence. Solvent extraction works for many plant parts, but because it is a lengthy and expensive process, it is used primarily when distillation is not an option.

Glossary

absolute: A highly concentrated floral essence obtained through the solvent extraction of flowers.

accord: A harmonic blend of certain fragrance notes. The most famous accord is the chypre type, a soft, honeylike melding of bergamot, oakmoss, sandalwood, patchouli, labdanum, jasmine, and rose.

aldehyde: A synthetic compound, produced by modern chemistry, that has a bold, clear note and diffuses well. Small amounts of aldehydes blended with natural scents give a fragrance sparkle, but larger amounts make it harsh.

bouquet: A perfume composed of many florals. The term also refers to the combined effect of the constituents of a fragrance.

concrete: A substance that consists of an essential oil solidified in plant paraffin. A concrete results when flowers undergo solvent extraction.

essential oil: A natural oil with a perceptible fragrance or flavor. Essential oils are volatile; that is, their molecules quickly evaporate and reach the odor receptors in the nose.

fixative: A perfume component with a high molecular weight, which lengthens the period that the perfume's odor can be perceived. Sandalwood, oakmoss, and orrisroot prolong the life of potpourri, and their oils do the same for perfume.

flacon: A perfume bottle. The term is adopted from the French word for "flask."

gas chromatography: A system whereby the components of an essential oil can be identified, allowing perfumers to reproduce scents. An essential oil is injected into a tube, which is then placed in a machine that analyzes and graphs the oil's component molecules and their proportions.

grand parfum: A top-of-the-line fragrance, created with great artistry and a high proportion of natural oils.

incense: A sweet-smelling smoke used for scenting a room or environment. There are two kinds of incense: One is a dried tree resin that is sprinkled on a hot brazier; the other a slow-burning stick form made from a paste of essential oils, vegetable gum, and aromatic sawdust.

note: An aspect of a perfume's range. The top note, for example, is the first impression a person has of a fragrance. This top note is of critical importance in marketing a fragrance because if the first experience is not pleasing, a customer will not be tempted to explore further. The middle or heart notes follow, as a perfume warms on the skin. And the base note, or dry-out note, is the scent that clings as long as the fragrance is perceptible. The molecules in a perfume that cling the longest are those that have the greatest molecular weight, such as components of sandalwood or musk. A fragrance might have top notes of lavender, middle notes of rose and violet, and a base note of sandalwood.

perfumer's alcohol: An ethyl alcohol made from grain, fruit, or other sources, used as a carrier for essential oils. A fragrance's source of alcohol can affect its character.

pomander: A perforated ball filled with aromatic ingredients such as spices, woods, and dried herbs and flowers.

potpourri: A bowl or jar filled with dried flowers and herbs that are rich in essential oils. During the seventeenth and eighteenth centuries, salt and water were sometimes added to potpourris to heighten the scent by introducing a mild fermentation.

sachet: A fabric pouch of dried herbs, flowers, and spices, often worn on the person.

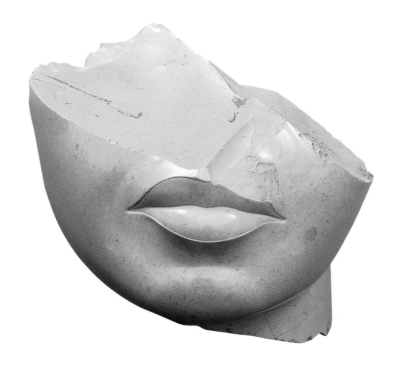

Scent in the
Fertile Crescent

❦━◆━❖━◆━❖━❦

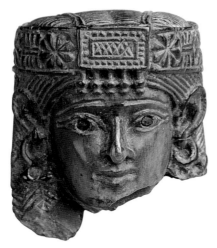

Scented oils were often used to add luster to the hair. In Mesopotamia, women wore their hair long and full. This ivory head of a woman was found at Nimrud, a capital of Assyria, and dates to the 8th century B.C.

Rogers Fund, 1954 54.117.8

On the previous page is a fragment of a yellow jasper head of an Egyptian queen, 5¹⁄₂ inches (14 cm) tall, from the 18th Dynasty, ca. 1353–1336 B.C.

Purchase, Edward S. Harkness Gift, 1926
26.7.1396
Photograph by Bruce White

THE AROMATICS OF THE ANCIENT NEAR EAST

The story of perfume begins with the birth of urban life in the ancient Near East some five thousand years ago. The word "perfume," from the Latin *per fumum*, means "through smoke," and the first perfumes were aromatics kindled as incense to gods and ancestors. Scented smoke was thought to attract good influences.

Burning incense was believed to connect humans with deities in the heavens by providing a means of carrying prayers aloft. It was also believed that incense's perfume was pleasing to the gods and that one's ancestors could derive sustenance from the fumes. For the Mesopotamians, the most prized of all incense varieties was the fragrant cedar of Lebanon (*Cedrus libani*). Vast quantities of the wood and resin of this tree were imported to Mesopotamia from the forests of Lebanon, far to the northwest. The ancient Akkadian word *lubbunu*, meaning "incense," still lingers in the word "Lebanon."

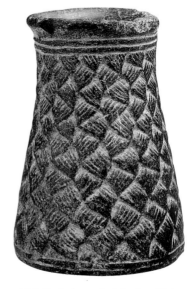

This little jar, only 3 inches (7.6 cm) tall, was carved out of steatite or chlorite, two stones found in the mountains of Iran. It was made sometime between 2750 and 2350 B.C., and may have once been used for perfumed oils or some type of cosmetic.

Purchase, Mrs. Vladimir S. Littauer Gift, 1970 1970.33.2

The resinous woods of pine, cypress, and fir trees were also burned in public ceremonies and private devotions. All of these woods possess a clean, refreshing scent. Although not a conifer, the evergreen myrtle shrub has a similar clean aroma that was enjoyed in incense.

Myrtle's fragrant, glossy leaves are deep green, somewhat like those of boxwood. (In the Near East many centuries later, hedges of aromatic myrtle would have an important place in formal Islamic gardens.) Juniper berries, familiar today as the source of the odor and flavor of gin, were also prized and used in incense.

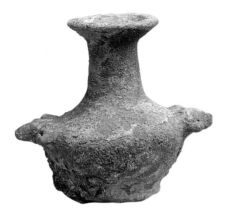

PERFUME FOR THE PERSON

Incense may have been the most commonly used aromatic product in the ancient Near East. However, it was not the only type of manufactured scent; perfume for the body was used as well. Collections of oil storage jars and tiny cosmetic containers, along with written records and perfume recipes dating to about 1750 B.C., have been excavated at

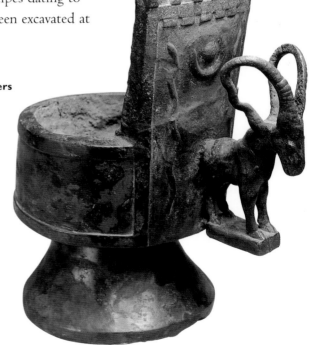

As early as the 2nd millennium B.C., cast-bronze cosmetic containers shaped like tiny vases and animals were made throughout the area of what is now southeastern Iran and Afghanistan. This little vase with ram's-head handles is just 4¹/₄ inches (10.8 cm) tall. The cosmetic stored inside would have been applied with the aid of a bronze stick, many of which were also designed with animal finials.

Gift of Sheldon Lewis Breithart, 1983   1983.535.36 A

Southern Arabia was the ancient world's center of trade for incense resins. Aromatics such as frankincense and myrrh reached the southern Levant (modern Israel and Jordan) and other trade destinations by land and sea routes. This Arabian bronze incense burner, which stands nearly 11 inches (28 cm) tall, was made in the 1st century B.C.

Gift of Dr. Sidney A. Charlat, in memory of his parents, Newman and Adele Charlat, 1949
49.71.2

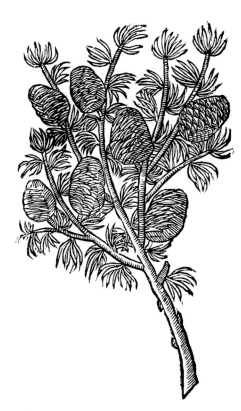

Fragrant wood and oil from the cedar of Lebanon, shown in the illustration above, provided the base for one of the world's first perfumes.

From *The Theatre of Plants, or an Herball of a Large Extent*, p. 1532, London, 1640
Gift of the Estate of Marie L. Russell, 1946 46.117.3

the palace ruins of the Syrian city of Mari. These jars and records also reveal that the palace had special rooms devoted to the blending of scented products and that both men and women served in the esteemed role of perfumer. Based largely on the resins and macerated leaves of pines and other conifers, Mari's perfume oils had fresh, pungent aromas that resembled those of the favored incenses.

THEN AND NOW

Like their counterparts in the ancient Near East, modern perfumers continue to draw from a great range of conifers when blending new perfumes and scenting soaps. Although the cedar of Lebanon is now endangered in the wild and its resin is no longer distilled, the leaves of its close relative *Cedrus atlantica*, from Morocco, are used in perfumery. Similarly, oils from the leaves of the western and eastern hemlocks, the black and the white spruces, and the balsam fir appear in modern toiletry products. Juniper berries, too, lend their brisk scent to colognes and chypre-type perfumes just as they did 4,000 years ago.

The people of the ancient Near East contributed to modern perfumery in several other areas as well. The Babylonians were the first to write herbals, recording the various properties and uses of plants, and they devised the earliest system of weights and measures for lightweight items, such as those used in perfumery. Even more importantly, in about 1400 B.C., craftsmen in the Near East discovered how to make glass. Knowledge of glassmaking techniques soon spread to Egypt, and by the mid–fourteenth century B.C., glass had become one of the choice materials for storing essential oils and perfumes.

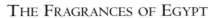

The playfulness that the ancient Egyptians brought to the luxury arts of makeup and beauty comes across in this 9-inch (22.9 cm) alabaster cosmetic spoon. Made in the 18th Dynasty in about 1400 B.C., it is carved in the form of a swimming girl towed by a gazelle. The body of the gazelle is hollowed out to form the bowl of the spoon. The girl's intricate coiffure and her narrow girdle are made of black slate.

Rogers Fund, 1926   26.2.47

The art of glassmaking was new to Egypt in the 18th Dynasty when this 6⁷/₈-inch (17.5 cm) bottle was made, ca.1353–1336 B.C. Along with stone and metal, glass would become one of the most familiar materials used for making toiletry items during this period. A wide variety of other Egyptian perfume bottles, cosmetic jars, and kohl tubes were made similarly to this one, with alternating bands of colorful opaque glass.

Purchase, Edward S. Harkness Gift, 1926   26.7.1176

THE FRAGRANCES OF EGYPT

Because of the wealth of written and pictorial records that have been preserved from ancient Egypt, far more is known about perfumery techniques and habits there than in Mesopotamia, on the other side of the Fertile Crescent. Over many centuries, the Egyptians exhibited a wonderful sense of play and experimentation in extracting scents from petals and leaves, and in concocting potions, beauty aids, and perfumes.

For the Egyptians (as for all cultures that preceded the development of alcohol in the fourteenth century), perfumes used on the body were made with an oil base; lotions and pomades often contained milk or honey as well as oil. Just as now, beauty lotions were credited with magical results. One promised to "banish wrinkles," another to "turn an old man into a youth," others simply to soften the skin. The harsh Egyptian sun could easily leave the skin dry and cracked, so it was essential that people keep themselves well-anointed with emollients.

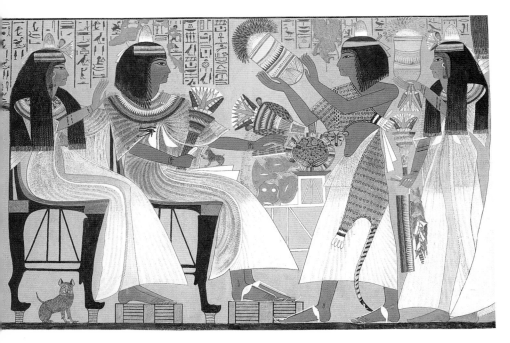

In this detail of a painting copied from one that dates to about 1275 B.C., in the Tomb of Ipuy, at Thebes, Ipuy and his wife and children wear perfumed cones on their heads.
Rogers Fund, 1930   30.4.114

To make the interior of this alabaster perfume bottle hollow, the vessel had to be made in two vertical halves, which were then cemented together. The inlay of a princess standing on a lotus flower was made with carnelian, obsidian, and colored glass. The 4¼-inch (10.8 cm) bottle dates to about 1340–1336 B.C.
Rogers Fund, 1940   40.2.4

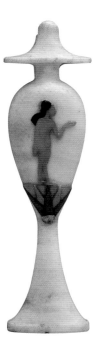

One noted method for keeping the skin oiled was to wear a molded cone of scented and solidified tallow on top of the head. In the heat of the day, the scent was released as the cone melted, covering the body with perfume and leaving the skin and hair glistening with oil. Perfumed cones are believed to have been worn when people attended feasts and festivals, and were used by men and women, royals and commoners alike.

Egyptian perfumers made their cones and other scented products by the maceration process. First a carrier of liquid fat or oil was made from purified tallow, olives, castor beans, linseed, safflower seed, radish seed, or lettuce seed. Then the carrier was heated with aromatic leaves, roots, bark, and resins until the scent was absorbed. Perfumers kept their specific blending techniques closely guarded secrets.

Because perfumed oils and lotions were costly, they were usually kept in small containers. Thus, Egyptian craftsmen produced cosmetic jars, pots, and boxes of enormous and exquisite variety. Many of these containers were fashioned from alabaster and other types of stone, which helped to keep the oils and fatty lotions cool.

For the fashion- and beauty-conscious Egyptians, cleanliness and care of the body were paramount. Priests were required to bathe three times a day. For many people of the upper classes, bathing was a daily ritual and was followed by pampering the body and applying beauty products. To make rouge, the Egyptians used a mortar and pestle to grind resins into a powder, which was then blended with animal or vegetable oils and red ocher, a natural pigment. A reddish-gold nail coloring was made by mixing the dried and powdered leaves and roots of the henna plant with water. Eye makeup known as kohl was made of antimony or charcoal ground fine on a small grindstone, then combined with water and powdered resin. It was applied around the eyelid with an applicator made of bone or hematite. In the desert today, Bedouin continue to wear kohl eye makeup, which is thought to reduce glare from the sun.

The names of Amenhotep III and Queen Sitamun are inlaid in black glaze on this 5⁵/₈-inch (14.3 cm) faience kohl tube. It was made in the form of a hollow reed, late in Dynasty 18, between 1391 and 1353 B.C.
Purchase, Edward S. Harkness Gift, 1926   26.7.910

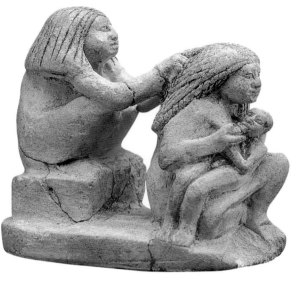

This tiny sculpture depicts a woman having her hair dressed while she nurses her child. Only 2⁷/₈ inches (7.3 cm) tall, it was made sometime between the 12th and 13th Dynasties, ca. 1991–1668 B.C. During this period, women frequently wore their hair parted in the middle and hanging to their shoulders or longer. On formal occasions women wore wigs, as did Egyptian men.
Rogers Fund, 1922   22.2.35

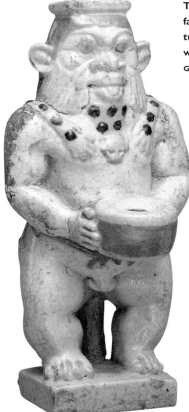

This figure with a leonine head is the Egyptian god **Bes**. He is shown here as a 3⅝-inch (9.2 cm) faience cosmetic container, made in Dynasty 27, 525–404 B.C. In his hands is the cap of a kohl tube, which has a small hole in the top for the insertion of an applicator. At one time the cap would have fit over a tube for the kohl (now missing), which could be detached for filling.
Gift of Norbert Schimmel Trust, 1989   1989.281.94

THE AROMA OF INCENSE

The attention paid to personal beauty in ancient Egypt was more than matched by ministrations to gods and goddesses. Every morning, along vast temple corridors, priests "awakened" statues of deities by passing a censer of burning incense under their nostrils. Thus fortified by their inhalations, the deities were prepared to receive the many requests of their devotees.

The word for incense, 'ntyw, appears early in Egyptian writing and would have included a variety of aromatic woods and resins. Two of the best-known incense resins were frankincense (*Boswellia papyrifera*) and myrrh (*Commiphora myrrha*), members of the bal-sam family. They were transported to Egypt from the land of Punt, or Pwenet, an area that is believed to be in what is now Somalia and northern Ethiopia. These African varieties are closely related to Arabian frankincense and myrrh, which were presented to the infant Jesus by the legendary Magi.

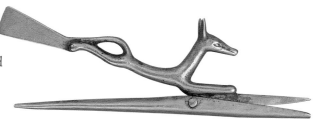

This delicate cosmetic implement, with its lively jackal decoration, was made during the early 18th Dynasty, in about 1550 B.C. Measuring only 3⅜ inches (8.6 cm) long, the tool is thought to have been used to curl hair. It was mechanically activated by a transverse pin located below the jackal's shoulder. This is the only known implement of its kind made of pure gold.
Purchase, Lila Acheson Wallace Gift, 1977   1977.169

Scent and flowers were important even in death in Egypt. This flower collar, 18¹/₂ inches (47 cm) wide, was worn by a guest at King Tutankhamen's funerary banquet at Thebes, about 1327 B.C., during the 18th Dynasty. It is made with a papyrus backing covered with rows of olive leaves, cornflowers, and woody nightshade berries, and is decorated with blue faience beads strung on strips of palm leaves. It was found in the embalmer's cache in the Valley of Kings.

Gift of Theodore M. Davis, 1909   09.184.216

Frankincense and myrrh were burned to mark a variety of ceremonies, such as coronations of pharaohs, openings of shrines, and passings of the dead. At funerals, the perfumed smoke was believed to guide the soul to heaven and to protect it from harmful influences. Vast quantities of scented resins were required for such ceremonies. By far the greatest effort to obtain them was made by Queen Hatshepsut, who reigned in the New Kingdom from about 1473 to 1458 B.C. Hatshepsut sent an army of soldiers and retainers to gather incense resins in Punt. Hatshepsut's workers not only gathered the dried resins in the usual way, by scraping them off the trees, but also dug up frankincense and myrrh trees, root ball and all, and carried them back to Hatshepsut's marvelous temple at Deir el Bahri. Details of the Egyptians' visit to the land of Punt and their transport of its trees were recorded in descriptive wall reliefs at the temple.

Queen Hatshepsut was often depicted as a male ruler, complete with beard. In the red-granite sculpture at right, 8 foot 7 inches (261.6 cm) tall, she is shown holding two offering jars. Hatshepsut had been the consort of King Tuthmosis II. When the king died in 1479 B.C., his son Tuthmosis III was too young to reign, and Hatshepsut became regent. Within a few years, however, she had contrived to have herself crowned king with full pharaonic powers. Her magnificent temple at Deir el Bahri, which this sculpture once adorned, was intended to legitimize and commemorate her rule.

Rogers Fund, 1929   29.3.1   Photograph by Schecter Lee

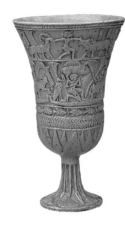

This blue-lotus faience chalice dates to the 22nd Dynasty, 945–715 B.C. The sepals of the lotus encircle the bowl of the cup; above them, the flower's watery habitat is depicted in miniature relief. This chalice was a religious object, symbolizing—like the fragrant flower itself—the eternal renewal of life in all its richness and variety.

Purchase, Edward S. Harkness Gift, 1926   26.7.971
Photograph by Schecter Lee

Hatshepsut was not the only one to enjoy fragrant plants. Favorites among the Egyptian public were cypress, juniper, sweet flag, lilies, and the white water lily (*Nymphaea lotus*). Favored above all was the blue lotus (*Nymphaea caerulea*), which has a sweet, almost fruity aroma. Despite its name, this blue flower is actually a water lily, a distant relative of the true lotus of Asia. The blue lotus was worn in the hair and carried in bouquets. The color of the petals evoked the heavens, with the golden center representing the sun disk of the god Amun-Ra. Just as the sun disappeared beneath the horizon, the blue lotus closed its petals until dawn.

The detail of a wall painting below depicts a canal in the Egyptian marshes. Holding a net between the two boats, fishermen haul in a good catch. Water lilies of two varieties are shown in full bloom along the top of the waterline. This painting is a copy of a mural in the Tomb of Ipuy, at Deir el Medina, Thebes. The original was painted in the 19th Dynasty in about 1275 B.C.

Rogers Fund, 1930   30.4.120

ISRAEL AND THE AROMATICS OF THE BIBLE

A garden inclosed is my sister, my spouse; a spring shut up, a fountain sealed.
Thy plants are an orchard of pomegranates, with pleasant fruits;
camphire, with spikenard, spikenard and saffron;
calamus and cinnamon, with all trees of frankincense;
myrrh and aloes, with all the chief spices.

Song of Solomon, 4:12–14

The Bible is a wonderful record of the imported and native scents that were favored in the ancient Near East and how they were used. Specifically, the Song

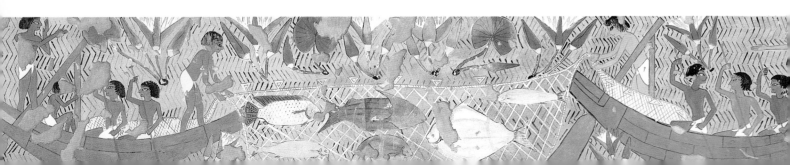

of Solomon ranks among the greatest of the world's aromatic verses. Even in the short passage above, many spices are mentioned, with many origins and uses.

The fragrant wood and oils of the camphire, or camphor, tree were imported from Asia. Spikenard comes from the root of the Indian plant *Nardostachys jatamansi*, a member of the valerian family. Its agreeably pungent scent was used most famously by Mary Magdalene to perfume the feet of Jesus.

Saffron is actually the stigma of the saffron crocus. Its clean, astringent scent was appreciated as a perfume by the Egyptians and Hebrews, although today saffron is used mainly as a flavoring in food. Calamus is the sweet flag, a rush with a cinnamonlike scent. The cinnamon of the Bible is the same spice used today in cooking and potpourris, and had to be imported to Israel from India.

Costly myrrh was used not only as an ingredient in incense but also in perfumes for the body. Esther 2:12–13 records the twelve-month period in which virgins were prepared for the harem of King Ahasuerus, "six months with oil of myrrh, and six months with sweet odors, and with other things for the purifying of the women."

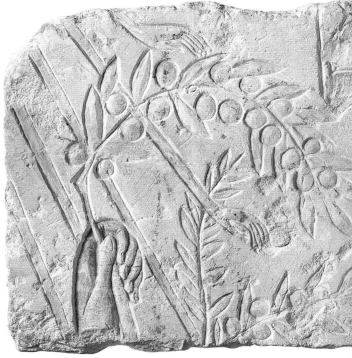

This detail of a painted limestone relief depicts the hand of the pharaoh Akhenaten holding an olive branch. Olive oil was one of the many types of oils and fats used as a base for perfumes throughout the Near East and the ancient Mediterranean region. In Egypt, sesame, linseed, and almond oils were also commonly used, as were animal fats. The relief fragment dates to about 1345–1335 B.C., during the 18th Dynasty.
Gift of Norbert Schimmel, 1981   1981.449

The aloes mentioned in the Song of Solomon is not *Aloe vera*, the aloe commonly used today as a skin salve, but *Aquilaria agallocha*, a tree that develops an exquisite scent only when infested by certain pathogens.

In China, the aloes is known as "sinking wood" because the pathogen damage increases the density of the wood to such an extent that it will sink in water. Incense made from aloes is still used in the Near East, where it is known as *oudh*, but it is reserved for important occasions because of its high cost.

OTHER FRAGRANCES

The Hebrews also imported frankincense, cinnamon, and balsam, and they grew their own fragrant myrtle, which is also mentioned throughout the Bible. Isaiah promised that "instead of the brier shall come up the myrtle tree" (Isaiah 55:13). Myrtle branches, along with pine boughs and olive branches, were used to make booths at the original Feast of the Tabernacles (Nehemiah 8:15). And the Hebrew word for "myrtle" is *hadas*, which is the root of "Hadassah," the Hebrew name of Queen Esther.

A darker aromatic episode is revealed in the story of the biblical heroine Judith. She is recorded as having removed her widow's dress, "washed all over, anointed herself with costly perfumes, dressed her hair, wrapped a turban around it, and put on the dress she used to wear on joyful occasions" (Judith, 10:3–5). Perfumed and adorned, Judith gained access to the tent of Holofernes and seduced and then slew him. Such is the power of scent.

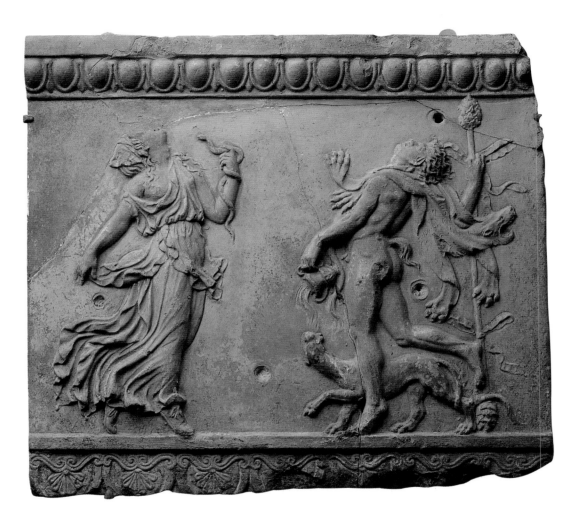

Scent in the
Classical World

❧⟶◦⟵❧

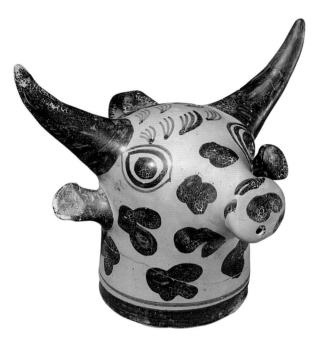

This terra-cotta vase, which might have held perfume, is only 3³/₄ inches (9.5 cm) tall and was made during the late Minoan period about 1450–1400 B.C.

Gift of Alastair B. Martin, 1973   1973.35

On the previous page is a Roman terra-cotta plaque with relief figures of a satyr and maenad, which dates to between 31 B.C. and A.D. 14.

Rogers Fund 1912   12.232.8 B
Photograph by Schecter Lee

THE PERFUMES OF CRETE

When a Minoan artist in about 1500 B.C. painted frescoes on the palace walls at Knossos, on the island of Crete, he depicted an elegant society. Women wore fine jewelry and stylish dresses, and they piled their hair into coils adorned with chains and strands of pearls. Men appeared equally fashion-conscious and proud of their athletic bodies. Minoan men and women also are known to have enjoyed making elaborate toilets—bathing, shaving, and anointing themselves with perfumed oils.

Minoan culture, which lasted from about 3000 to 1100 B.C., had contacts with Egypt and Greece. In the late Minoan period, ships brought Egyptian luxury goods to Crete and the island of Cyprus as well. Island residents in turn loaded the ships with aromatic oils that were sent to the Near East, Phoenicia, and Egypt. Favorite perfumery scents among the Minoans included rose and lily. A fresco dating from about 1719 B.C at Knossos includes a representation of two roses, *Rosa gallica* and *Rosa phoenicia*. And a carved stela from 2000 B.C. bears the following inscription:

> The lily carved here is the scented symbol
> of Seka, who in life emanated only perfume.

GREEK AROMATICS

As civilization flourished on Crete, centers of culture grew on the Greek mainland as well. But during three centuries of intense disruption and warfare on the mainland—from about 1200 to 900 B.C.— artistic creativity all but ceased.

However, by the seventh century B.C., the cities of Athens and Corinth had once again begun blending and exporting oils perfumed with macerated rose, lily, iris, sage, thyme, marjoram, mint, and anise. And by that date, the people of Greece themselves were wearing scented oils and pomades as well, as evidenced in the following quotation from Homer's *The Iliad*:

> Here first she bathes; and round her body pours
> Soft oils of fragrance, and ambrosial show'rs.

Terra-cotta perfume containers were produced as an industry in Corinth, and they were made in other cities as well. Greek craftsmen were masters at creating decorated bottles and jars for cosmetics of all kinds. One type was the *pyxis*, a covered box often elaborated with detailed painted decoration. Another container, the *alabastron*, was designed as an elongated vial with a rounded bottom and a small opening on top. A third type, the *aryballos*, came in a great variety of shapes, from small jugs to amusing and beautiful animal and human forms.

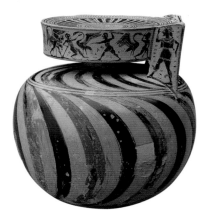

The 3 1/16-inch (7.7 cm) terra-cotta *aryballos* at left, made in about 570 B.C., was signed by its maker, **Nearchos**, who may have painted it as well. A similar *aryballos* hangs from the youth's wrist on the detail of the grave marker above, which dates to about 540 B.C.

Aryballos: Purchase, The Cesnola Collection, by exchange, 1926   26.49
Photograph by Schecter Lee
Grave marker: Frederick C. Hewitt, Rogers, and Munsey Funds, 1911, 1921, 1936, and 1938; and Anonymous Gift, 1951
11.185

In ancient Greece, a covered box made to hold cosmetics and other toiletries was called a *pyxis*. The footed example at right is made of terra-cotta and stands 6¾ inches (17.1 cm) tall. The decoration, attributed to the Penthesilea Painter, tells the tale of the judgment of Paris. In the story, Paris was tending his flocks on Mount Ida when he was asked to decide which of three goddesses was the fairest. This view of the *pyxis* shows two of the goddesses: Athena, carrying her helmet and spear, and Hera, wearing a veil. Ultimately, Paris chose the third goddess, Aphrodite (not visible here). This jar was made in about 460 B.C. in the Attic region of Greece, in what is now the area of Athens.

Rogers Fund, 1907   07.286.36

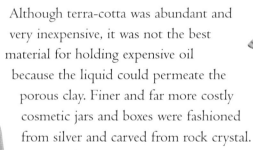

Although terra-cotta was abundant and very inexpensive, it was not the best material for holding expensive oil because the liquid could permeate the porous clay. Finer and far more costly cosmetic jars and boxes were fashioned from silver and carved from rock crystal.

By the sixth century B.C., perfumes and other beauty products had become very popular among the Greeks. Women accentuated their eyes with kohl, wore rouge, lightened their complexions with white-lead powder, and were known to bleach

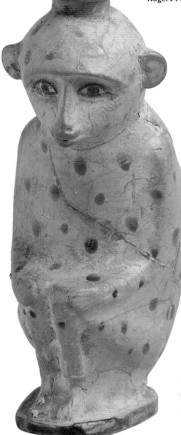

Cosmetic containers made in the forms of animals, including monkeys and baboons, were first fashioned in Egypt, but this 3⅝-inch (9.2 cm) terra-cotta monkey was made in Greece in the first quarter of the 6th century B.C. The flat lip surrounding the neck of Greek perfume vessels allowed for the careful pouring of precious oils. Like other perfume vases, this one could be refilled with oils at home or in a perfume shop. In ancient Greece, perfume shops were social gathering places, where news and gossip were exchanged.

Purchase, Sandra Brue Gift, 1992   1992.11.2

This 6¼-inch (15.9 cm) bird-shaped bottle, made in the city of **Corinth** in the 7th century B.C., is one of the great variety of figural perfume bottles manufactured in that city. Like this one, many Greek perfume vessels were designed to be carried by straps or cords rather than to sit flat on a tabletop.

Rogers Fund, 1947   47.100.2
Photograph by Schecter Lee

The remarkable faience *aryballos* at right (shown in two views) is only 2⅛ inches (5.4 cm) tall. It consists of four heads: two large ones depicting a young woman with long hair and a shrieking demon, and two smaller ones of a roaring lion and an African youth with fanglike teeth. It is possible that this *aryballos* may not have served as an ordinary perfume flask but as a receptacle for a medicinal substance with mind-altering properties. The main centers of faience perfume-container production were on the island of **Rhodes** and in the **Nile Delta** region during the late 6th and early 5th centuries B.C.

Classical Purchase Fund, 1992 1992.11.59
Photograph by Schecter Lee

their hair. Both men and women smoothed perfumed creams and oils on their skin and sprinkled themselves with herbal- and floral-scented waters. But not everyone wore or appreciated perfume. The Athenian statesman Solon tried to ban its use, claiming that it represented the corrupt and luxurious lifestyle of Persia, Greece's traditional enemy.

AROMATICS OF THE EAST

The Persian influence on Greek life grew after Alexander the Great and his armies conquered Egypt and the Persian empire in the fourth century B.C. Among the "orientalizing" influences that appeared at that time were an increased use of perfumes and incense, and a greater awareness of exotic fragrance plants. Alexander himself sent seeds and cuttings of Persian plants to his teacher in Athens, Theophrastus, who created a botanical garden and wrote the world's first treatise on scent, *Concerning Odors*. The text included

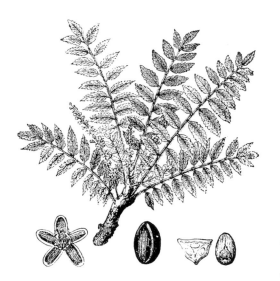

Frankincense, illustrated at left, was beloved by the Egyptians and Persians, and was used as an incense in Greece. Alexander the Great sent exploratory missions in search of plants throughout the Near East. Their findings were later recorded by Theophrastus of Athens: "The trees of frankincense and myrrh grow partly in the mountains, and partly on private estates at the foot of the mountains. . . . The frankincense tree, it is said, is not tall, about five cubits high, and is much branched."

From *The Book of Perfumes*, by Eugene Rimmel, London, 1865
The Metropolitan Museum of Art, Thomas J. Watson Library

an inventory of all the Greek and imported aromatic plants known at the time. It also discussed the ways in which aromatics could be artfully blended by the perfumer.

Theophrastus outlined the use of dried flowers and herbs, the shelf life of scented products, the suitability of various perfumes for states of mind and health, and the properties of various oils that might be used as carriers of scent. "The lightest [perfumes] are rose-perfume and kypros, which seem to be the best suited to men, as also is lily-perfume," Theophrastus wrote. "The best for women are myrrh-oil, megaleion [a blend of balsam, cassia, resins, and other aromatics], the Egyptian, sweet marjoram, and spikenard: for these

This finely decorated terra-cotta vessel was made in Greece in the late 7th century B.C. and is 3 1/8 inches (7.9 cm) tall. The ram's head that tops the vessel can be removed and may have once held an applicator for cosmetics.

Classical Purchase Fund, 1977   1977.11.3
Photograph by Schecter Lee

owing to their strength and substantial character do not easily evaporate and are not easily made to disperse, and a lasting perfume is what women require."

When Alexander died in 323 B.C., he was cremated in Babylon on a pyre laden with frankincense and myrrh. Rule of Alexander's empire was divided among his generals. Egypt and Libya were taken over by Ptolemy I, who established a dynasty of rulers based in Alexandria, the most famous and wealthy of the successor states. The beautiful Cleopatra (69–30 B.C.) was the fifteenth and last of the Ptolemies. She wanted to unite Egypt with the rising power of Rome through her lover, the Roman orator and soldier Marc Antony.

When Cleopatra went to meet Antony at sea, it was as the goddess Venus traveling across the water in human form. Cleopatra herself was

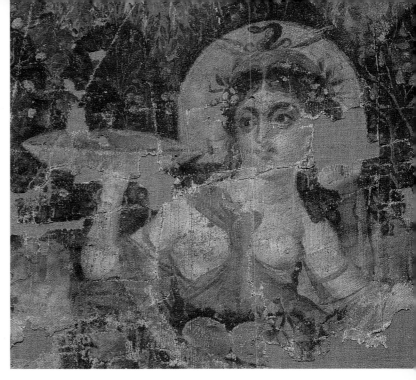

This intriguing detail of a painting fragment depicts Euthenia in a garden. It was painted in Egypt in the 1st century B.C., when Egyptian rule had passed from Greece to Rome, and Egyptian concepts of beauty reflected the two influences. Along with scenting their bodies, upper-class Greek and Roman women took particular care of their complexions. Many went to bed wearing beauty masks blended from such ingredients as flour, honey, and egg white, which they washed off with milk or water in the morning.
Purchase, Mr. and Mrs. Nathaniel Spear Jr. Gift, 1984   1984.178

The design of cosmetic containers had changed quite a bit by the time this *pyxis* was made, in the 3rd century B.C. It was found in Italy near Orvieto, which was an Etruscan city. Shaped like a tent, the *pyxis* is worked in silver, chased with fine detail, and partially gilded. A small box such as this might have held emollient lotions, but not all of them were meant for use in this world. This *pyxis* is inscribed with the phrase "for the tomb."
Rogers Fund, 1903   03.24.6 A-B

This *amphoriskos,* or perfume vase, 6 inches (15.2 cm) tall, is one of a collection of silver cosmetic implements made in Etruria in the 3rd century B.C. The chased swag across the vase's middle section and the leaf design at its base give the vessel an especially elegant look. The sophisticated civilization that the Etruscans built in central Italy included twelve cities. They traded extensively with Greece and the East and became noted for their own works of art, including finely crafted jewelry as well as hollow vessels such as this one, in silver and gold.

Rogers Fund, 1903 03.24.5

anointed with the choicest rose-scented oils, and the sails of her ship were perfumed as well. On the ship's deck, incense burners exuded clouds of scent around her throne. Cleopatra's dream of uniting Egypt and Rome ultimately was not to be realized, but it was not for want of trying.

THE AROMA OF ROME

Long before Rome was established and civilized, the Etruscans had developed a vibrant culture in central Italy, in the region that is now Tuscany and Umbria. The Etruscans were fine metalsmiths and craftsmen and traded actively with cultures to the south and in the Near East. Etruscan perfumers used imported incense resins in their products, but they also made their own aromatic oils scented with myrtle, Spanish broom, rock rose, and pine— all Mediterranean plants.

There was little use for perfume or cosmetics of any kind in early Rome, but as contacts with the Etruscans, Phoenicians, and Greeks expanded over time, Roman use of scents and toiletries gradually increased as well. By the second century B.C., a

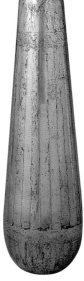

This *alabastron* was made in the late 5th or early 4th century B.C. At 8¼ inches (21 cm) long, it is one of the largest examples known in silver. Far more commonly, *alabastra* were fashioned from molded and modeled terra-cotta, carved alabaster, or blown glass. A gilt star rosette with twenty points radiates from the bottom of this *alabastron,* and a similar pattern appears at the top. Other Greek vessels exhibit a similar use of gilding in a striped design.

Classical Purchase Fund, 1994
1994.113

trickle of frankincense and myrrh, brought by ship from southern Arabia or from Alexandria, was making its way into Roman temples.

Roman enjoyment of incense and personal scents remained modest during the time of the early republic, but during the imperial period the city's use of scents exceeded all known limits. Rome's great consumption of frankincense and myrrh during this period created balance-of-payment problems for the empire.

In the first century A.D., an estimated five hundred tons of myrrh and twenty-five hundred tons of frankincense were exported from southern Arabia to Rome, where incense was used at all important state and religious ceremonies. Pliny the Elder recorded that the emperor Nero burned an entire year's growth of frankincense at the funeral of the empress Poppaea, in A.D. 65.

PERFUMERS OF ROME

In the shops of ancient Rome, perfume makers, called *aromatarii*, sold unguents in *buccheri*, or terra-cotta jars, and dispensed oils and scented wines in blown-glass flacons. The luxury-loving Romans had advanced the art of glassmaking and were masters of the art of blowing glass.

This Etruscan incense burner, made of cast bronze and standing 10⅝ inches (27 cm) tall, was fashioned in the late 6th or early 5th century B.C. Implements incorporating human figures were as popular in Etruria as they were in Greece. This woman wears a chiton, pointed shoes, and a veil that is gathered at the top of her head in the Etruscan style.

Gift from the Family of Howard J. Barnet, in his memory, 1992 1992.262

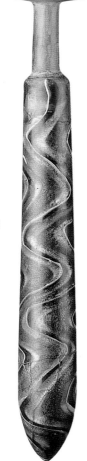

The craft of glass-blowing was invented in the 1st century B.C. It allowed glassworkers to create thin-walled vessels that were far more transparent than earlier glass as well as being watertight and nonreactive to oils and acids. This glass and gold-leaf *alabastron*, 7⅛ inches (18.1 cm) long, gets its shimmering effect through the fusing of glass rods of various colors. The top of the vessel can be removed to facilitate filling it with oil. The flask would have been kept upright by placing it on a metal tripod. At the perfumer's workshop, vessels of this shape were inserted in a shelf drilled with holes.

Gift of J. Pierpont Morgan, 1917
17.194.286
Photograph by Schecter Lee

The famous baths of Rome were among the places where perfume products were regularly used. In the fourth century A.D., the city of Rome had eleven public baths and more than eight hundred and fifty private baths. The public baths functioned as social centers; some were able to serve close to two thousand people.

Many of the perfumes and unguents that the Romans enjoyed were applied after they had immersed themselves in three bathing pools, each housed in a different room of the public bath. These were the *tepidarium*, the *caldarium*, and the *frigidarium*, or the tepid, hot, and cold rooms. Slaves called *cosmetae* prepared scents for Roman matrons, who made abundant use of creams, rouges, hair dyes, and cosmetics. Some Romans used a different scented unguent for each part of the body, even perfuming the soles of their feet.

Rome's perfumers used many aromatics from Italy and the eastern Mediterranean, including rose, sweet flag, iris, narcissus, saffron, and oakmoss. Because of the empire's extensive trade network, perfumers could also concoct blends with cinnamon, cardamom, nutmeg, ginger,

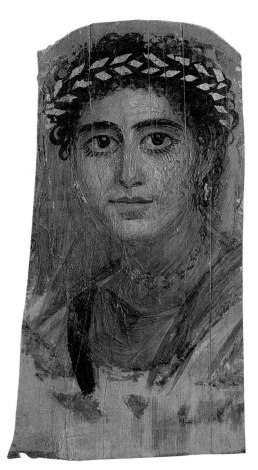

Roman ideals of feminine beauty are captured in this portrait of a woman. It was painted during the Roman period in Egypt, probably during the reign of Antonius Pius, between 138 and 161. Roman women lightened their skin and used kohl to accent their eyes, as did women throughout the classical world.

Rogers Fund, 1909 09.181.6

The *Rosa gallica* was known to the Roman scholar Pliny the Elder, who described it as "the rose of a hundred petals." The flower was later used to hybridize the *Rosa x damascena*, shown in the illustration below.

From *The Theatre of Plants, or an Herball of a Large Extent*, p. 1017, London, 1640
Gift of the Estate of Marie L. Russell, 1946   46.117.3

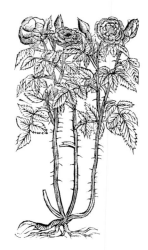

aloeswood and spikenard. Pliny recorded the wealth of aromatics in his *Natural History,* and two of the great physicians of the Roman era, Galen and Dioscorides, explored aromatics' medical possibilities.

The people of Rome loved the rose the most of all the flowers and spices, and they created the feast of Rosalia to honor it. Romans adorned themselves with roses at banquets; they decorated their villas with the flower; and on the occasion of a victory, they scattered roses through the streets. The emperor Nero once used four million sesterces' (about one hundred thousand dollars') worth of roses at one celebration, where a guest was asphyxiated by a cascade of roses. Extensive rose plantations were maintained in the nearby Campania region, but Rome's rose consumption was so great that additional plantations had to be established in Egypt as well.

Rome made several lasting contributions to the perfume industry. The empire's voracious consumption of perfume stimulated the creation of trade

The goddesses known in Greek mythology as the three Graces were an appropriate subject for a toiletry article. The goddesses appear in repoussé on the back of this Roman gilded-bronze mirror, made in the 2nd century A.D. The Greek name for the three Graces, "Charites," carries the meaning of charm, beauty, and favor, and it also expressed feelings of goodwill and gratitude. As divinities who were believed to foster fertility, the Graces were the object of cults in Greece and Asia Minor (now Turkey). In mythology they performed the role of handmaidens to Aphrodite, goddess of beauty and love. In early Greek art the Graces were shown fully clothed. This composition of the three nude figures was probably invented in the late Hellenistic period, or 1st century B.C. It later became the most commonly used formula for depicting the Graces.

Purchase, Sarah Campbell Blaffer Foundation Gift, 1987   1987.11.1

routes to Arabia, India, and even China; and its need for perfume containers gave glassmaking an unprecedented boost. In Rome, glass was used more often than clay, stone, or metal in making containers that held scent.

ALCHEMY AND SCENT

In the second century A.D., while Rome still ruled Egypt, important advancements toward modern perfumery came about through the development of alchemy in the city of Alexandria. Searching for knowledge, alchemy's early practitioners—Jewish mystics, Egyptian technologists, and Greek philosophers—examined all sorts of natural materials in hope of understanding how nature works and of discovering a divine spark or spirit that could be extracted.

Experiments were conducted in attempts to distill the "spirit" from plants and minerals, by submitting them to heat in water baths. An Alexandrian alchemist known to history as Maria the Prophetess (or Maria the Jewess) is credited with inventing the first still, which the alchemists used to distill oils from plants. Fragrant leaves and petals were placed in the still with water and then heated over a fire. Plant oils were released into the water as it simmered. The vaporized oil and water collected on the still's lid and were siphoned into a collecting vessel. Because oil and water do not mix, the plant oils could then be separated from the water.

It would be centuries before the process was perfected, but Maria's homely still, probably adapted from cooking pots, was the ancestor of the gleaming stainless-steel-and-glass retorts used in modern perfumery.

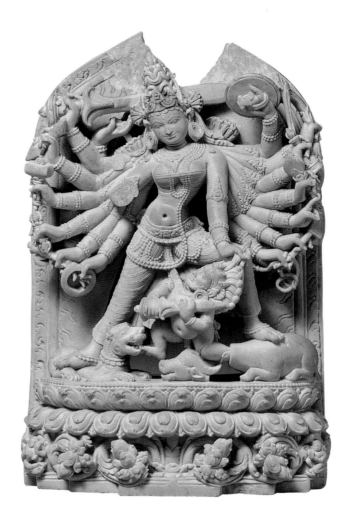

Scent in the East

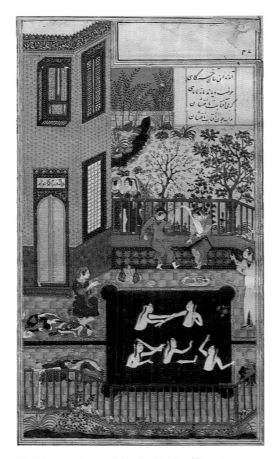

Bathing was key to Islamic rituals of beauty. Above, nymphs bathe in a garden in an illustration from a 1420s book, *Haft Paikar*, by Nizami.

Gift of Alexander Smith Cochran, 1913   13.228.13

On the previous page is a 5³/₈-inch (13.7 cm) figure of Durgā Mahishasuramardini. It was carved from argalite in India during the 12th century.

Purchase, Diana and Arthur G. Altschul Gift, 1993   1993.7

FRAGRANCES OF THE ISLAMIC WORLD

The thought of Islamic culture readily conjures up the scents of gardens, incense, and spices. The Islamic world has always appreciated the beauty of scent, and indeed, it has had a key role in the history of perfumery. With the fall of Rome in the fifth century, Arab and Persian scholars preserved the cultural achievements of the West and advanced the study of chemistry. A host of pharmacists, chemists, distillers, and medical writers flourished in the classical period of Islamic science. One of the most famous was Jabir ibn Hayyan (ca. 721–815), known to the West as Geber, who left an encyclopedia of general knowledge, of which several chapters discuss distillation. Another was Ar-Razi (ca. 840–924), an herbalist and physician of Baghdad who recorded experiments in distillation.

Equally important to perfumery was the Islamic world's expertise in trade. Through their vast networks, Arab and Persian merchants made spices from isolated areas of Asia available to the cultures of the Mediterranean.

People of Islam incorporated scent into their lives in many ways, including the use of incense. This incense burner, at 36 inches (91.4 cm) tall, is one of the stateliest of all Islamic bronze animals. Its form expresses the power of the dynamic Seljuqs, who controlled much of the Near East from the late 10th to the late 13th centuries.

Rogers Fund, 1951   51.56
Photograph by Schecter Lee

The prophet Muhammad said that the things he loved most in the world were "women, children, and perfumes." His beliefs and the religion of Islam that emerged from them in the early seventh century were congenial to merchants and trade. Cities along the trade routes protected caravans carrying spices and goods, and provided caravansaries—travelers' inns—for the traders, their attendants, and their animals. The "spices" that the caravans transported included pepper, cloves, resins such as frankincense and myrrh, and syrups flavored with roses and violets. By the ninth century, Muslim traders reached the coastal ports of China, and the scents of East Asia— orange, camphor, and musk—also became part of the culture of the Islamic world.

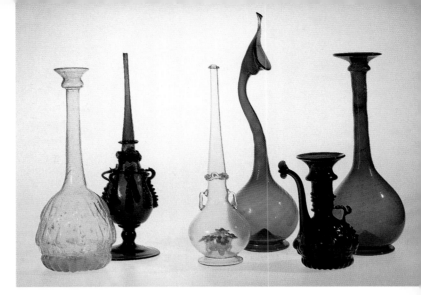

The making of beautiful glass may be counted among the outstanding achievements of Islamic artists, and perfume bottles have been a specialty. These Iranian bottles were made in the 19th century. The fourth bottle from left is a *gulabdan*, used for sprinkling rose water. The clear bottle next to it has glass flowers in its base.
Gift of Henry G. Marquand, 1883; Edward C. Moore Collection, Bequest of Edward C. Moore, 1891; and Gift of J. Pierpont Morgan, 1917. Left to right: 83.7.227, 83.7.260, 91.1.1554, 91.1.1557, 91.1.1600, 17.190.829

SCENTS OF EVERYDAY LIFE

Scents were worked into the tissue of everyday life in Islamic culture. Incense was burned in braziers in homes, in palaces, and in desert tents. The aroma of incense was always present at ceremonies for weddings and births. Of all the perfumery scents, the most prevalent was rose. The residents of Baghdad used some thirty thousand

Muslim craftspeople mastered glassblowing early on. This elegant 10¼-inch (26 cm) perfume sprinkler was made in Syria in the 12th century. When shaken, it dispensed drops of expensive perfume suspended in a heavy oil. Originally, the glass was clear with a greenish tint. Its present iridescence —an accidental but beautiful phenomenon—is due to its having been buried for many years.
Purchase, Richard S. Perkins Gift, 1977 1977.164

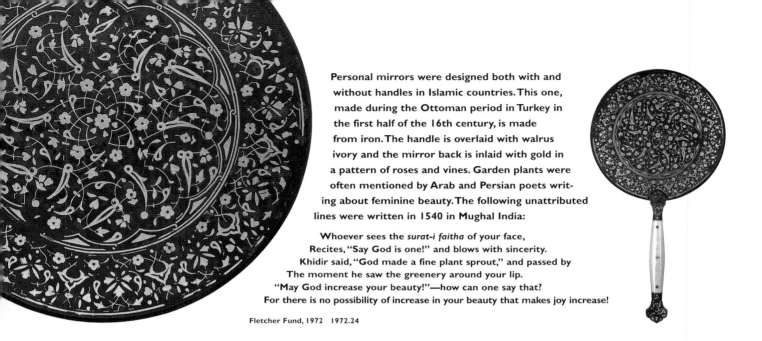

Personal mirrors were designed both with and without handles in Islamic countries. This one, made during the Ottoman period in Turkey in the first half of the 16th century, is made from iron. The handle is overlaid with walrus ivory and the mirror back is inlaid with gold in a pattern of roses and vines. Garden plants were often mentioned by Arab and Persian poets writing about feminine beauty. The following unattributed lines were written in 1540 in Mughal India:

Whoever sees the *surat-i faitha* of your face,
Recites, "Say God is one!" and blows with sincerity.
Khidir said, "God made a fine plant sprout," and passed by
The moment he saw the greenery around your lip.
"May God increase your beauty!"—how can one say that?
For there is no possibility of increase in your beauty that makes joy increase!

Fletcher Fund, 1972   1972.24

bottles of attar—oil of rose—each year. Rose oil was used on the skin and hair, and rose water was used as a flavoring for sherbets and the confection called *lokum*, known to the West as Turkish delight. On entering someone's home, a guest was sprinkled with rose water from a flask called a *gulabdan*.

Rose oil and rose water are the two products that result when rose petals are distilled and the oil separates—but not wholly—from the distilling water. In the past, much of the attar of rose used in the Islamic world was produced in the Syrian town of Al-Munazzah (modern al-Mizza). Today the most sought-after attar comes from Bulgaria's Kazanluk, the Valley of the Roses, where a Turkish merchant introduced the flower. Protected by mountains, this temperate region nurtures perfect rose oils that fetch astronomical prices. Jean Patou's Joy is characterized by a note of Bulgarian rose, *Rosa × damascena*, which is named after the city of Damascus.

Musk, a tenaciously sweet-scented oil that comes from a gland of the musk deer, had to be imported from China or northern India but was very popular as well. The Persian poet Firdausi declared that the houris, beautiful maidens of paradise, exuded the perfume of musk.

A POETIC SENSE OF FLOWERS

One of the great charms of Islamic culture lies in its praise for flowers. Tradition has it that the rose was created from a single drop of Muhammad's sweat as he ascended to the heavens on al-Buraq, his half-human, half-horse mount. Hafiz and Sa'di, two great Sufi poets of Iran, frequently praised the rose in their works, and indeed, one of Sa'di's greatest poems is the "Gulistan" ("Garden of Roses").

Many flowers have a special meaning for the Sufis, who suggest a setting of a rose garden for the practices of meditation and teaching. To them, the rose's perfume exudes the cry of "Allah! Allah!" The narcissus, with its white "eye," teaches the Sufis not to be blind to the divine glory present in the world. And the violet, which

This 4-inch (10.2 cm) glass perfume bottle, or *mukhula*, made in the 10th century, once held a floral-scented oil. Even today, many Arab perfumers prefer an oil base to alcohol, because oil "fixes" the scent better, meaning that it makes the scent last longer. The bright turquoise color of the bottle has long been favored in ceramics and glasswork in the Near East. When the bottle was made, a lustrous paint was used to create a geometric design over the turquoise background.
Gift of Helen Miller Gould, 1910   10.130.2649

In the image below, the prophet Muhammad rises to the heavens on the back of al-Buraq, though the drop of sweat that turned into the rose is not visible. The illustration is a leaf from a book called the *Bustan (Garden of Perfume)* by Sa'di, copied by the calligrapher Sultan-Muhammad Nur in 1514 and painted in central Asia in about 1520.
Purchase, Louis V. Bell Fund and The Vincent Astor Foundation Gift, 1974
1974.294.2

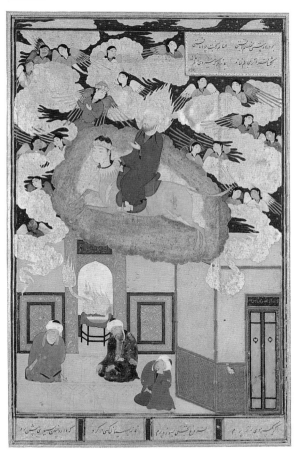

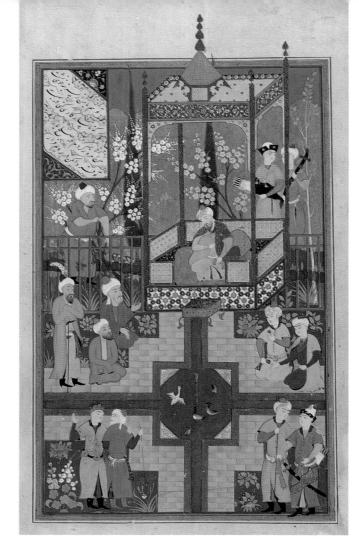

appears to bow down like the faithful at prayer, is a reminder of the virtue of adoration.

The black coloration deep inside the tulip demonstrates to the Sufis that the flower loved God so much that it burned its core to a cinder. To them, the hyacinth was the flower of Nowruz, the Persian New Year, celebrated on the spring equinox. In one of his poems, Hafiz described how he went into the market but, having very little money, passed the bakers' stalls by and instead bought a hyacinth "to feed his soul."

Tulips and hyacinths, whose bulbs were eventually exported to Europe and China, originated in the highlands of Iran and Anatolia. Planted in Persian gardens, their scents mingled with those of roses, jasmine, orange blossoms, and the fragrant leaves of myrtle. Contained within walls, the flowering plants, the sweet scents, and the sounds of trickling water and birdsong in Persian gardens were meant to emulate a paradise on earth.

In Persia, private gardens were paved enclosures in which water was as important as the plants. A typical garden, such as the one above, included a small central pool and channels of water that divided the garden into quarters, an allusion to the four corners of the earth. This illustration is from an early-16th-century copy of a 13th-century text, the *Bustan* by Sa'di. In it, the king of Syria is shown sitting in his garden in the spring, conversing with paupers.

Frederick C. Hewitt Fund, 1911   11.134.2

IN AN INDIAN GARDEN

Babur (1483–1530), the first Mughal ruler of India, was steeped in the Persian love of flowers and gardens. He introduced the Persian garden style to India and wrote that "from the excellencies of its sweet-smelling flowers, one may prefer the fragrances of India to those of the flowers of the whole world. It has so many that nothing in the universe can be compared to them."

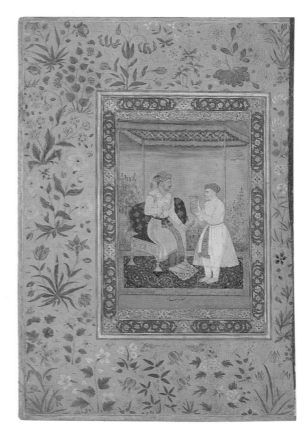

Babur's descendant the emperor Jahangir restored an ancient Hindu garden in Kashmir with his favorite wife, Nur Jahan. They called it Shalimar (Abode of Love) and filled it with roses, carnations, orange trees, cedars, and narcissi. Shalimar also became known as Farah-baksh (Bestower of Bliss) and over its entrance were inscribed the following words: "If indeed there is a paradise upon earth, it is here, it is here, it is here." Small wonder that this garden became the inspiration for one of the most famous of twentieth-century perfumes.

Jahangir, who created the garden Shalimar, is shown at right, sitting in his garden with his vizier. This page, painted by the artist Manohar in the mid–17th century, the Mughal period, is from an album assembled for Jahangir's son Shah Jahan. The elaborate perfume flask above left, 2½-inches (6.4 cm) tall, also dates from mid-17th-century India. The flask is carved from rock crystal in the shape of a mango and is set with gold, enamel, rubies, and emeralds. Artists of this period loved to combine natural forms with precious materials.

Painting: Purchase, Rogers Fund and The Kevorkian Foundation Gift, 1955 55.121.10.23
Flask: Purchase, Mrs. Charles Wrightsman Gift, 1993 1993.18

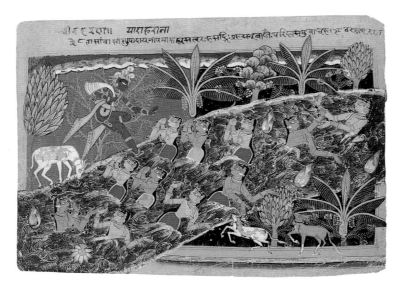

The rituals of beauty—bathing and anointing with perfumed oils—have been part of Indian culture for centuries. The bathing scene above is a famous one. This version of the scene was painted in about 1560 as a page in the *Bhagavata Purana*. In it, bathing women stand up to plead with the blue-skinned god Krishna to return their clothing, which he has stolen.

Gift of H. Rubin Foundation, Inc., 1972   1972.260
Photograph by Schecter Lee

THE PERFUMES OF INDIA

Babur's assessment of the wealth of flowers and fragrances in India was correct. The country possesses a vast range of climatic conditions, from humid jungles to Himalayan meadows. Thus aromatic plants have always been available for perfumery and pharmacy, and the customs of the early cultures of India freely encouraged lavish use of botanical products. As the religions of the Jains, the Buddhists, and the Brahmins developed, they all encouraged frequent bathing and ritual washings; fragrant oils, powders, and pastes were added to the body after these cleansings.

One Sanskrit author offered advice on providing pleasures of the daily bath for different types of bathers. For a king's bath, he prescribed that beautiful attendants should pour warm water on the king's body, wash his hair and scalp with the pulp of a fragrant fruit called *amalaka,* and then rinse the hair clean. For athletes, the author recommended that after bathing and drying, the athletes' bodies be massaged with a fragrant oil by female attendants. The massage oil used in postbath rituals was a complex blend of sesame oil perfumed with jasmine, coriander, cardamom, basil, costus, pandanus, agarwood, pine, saffron, champac, and clove. (The Indians not only gave and received perfumed rubdowns themselves but also gave the female elephant one that was expected to inflame the male elephant to passion—an elephant aphrodisiac.)

This mid-13th-century carved-stone relief depicts a female figure known as a *shalabanjika* holding a branch from a fragrant plant in her hand. The outside of a temple was usually covered with many relief sculptures such as this one, which is thought to have come from the Surya Temple at Konorak. A temple was often envisioned as the central axis of the world, in the form of a mountain inhabited by a god. The temple itself was therefore worshiped.

Rogers Fund, 1965 65.108
Photograph by Schecter Lee

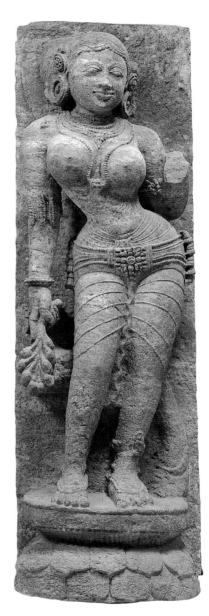

The *Kama Sutra*, written in about the year 400, speaks of scent in the erotic embraces that were supposed to mirror the union of the deity and the soul. "The Ritusanhara," a Sanskrit poem, also describes scent's allure:

> With their soft hips covered with beautiful fabrics and wrappings, their breasts perfumed with sandalwood, covered with necklaces and jewels, and with hair perfumed from the bath, the beautiful women coax their lovers to burning desire.

The Indian perfumer was known as the *gandhika*, or "scenter," who plied his trade amid fragrant heaps of spices and herbs. These aromatics would be ground into powders or macerated with oils for cosmetics. One special technique was to embed jasmine flowers in sesame seeds until they absorbed the jasmine scent. The flowers were then sifted out and the oil pressed from the sesame seeds. The most important use of the oil was for dressing the hair, which would exude the jasmine scent for a long time afterward.

INDIAN AROMATICS

There are many scents that are associated specifically with India, but sandalwood has perhaps the strongest connection. It is a crime to fell a sandalwood tree anywhere in India without government authorization, and the

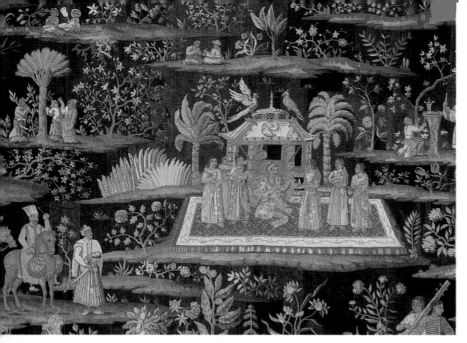

India's wealth of perfume and spice materials was acknowledged around the world. The scene above, depicting India's flowers, fruit trees, and other plants, is a detail from an English tapestry designed about 1690 and probably woven by John Vanderbank sometime before 1715.

Gift of Mrs. George F. Baker, 1953   53.165.1

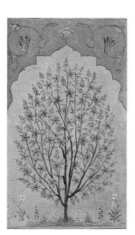

In Mughal India, the concept of perfume was more than just scent applied to the body. Flowering trees, which perfumed the air, were an important part of the design of gardens, where God was seen as the great master painter. As one Mughal poet wrote:

> Before the wise the green leaves of the trees
> Are each a page from the book
> of the Creator's wisdom.

The flowering tree in its gilded garden setting, left, is a detail from a page of a 17th-century album of paintings, poetry, and calligraphy that was once part of a royal library in India.

Bequest of Cora Timken Burnett, 1956   57.51.34

Mysore area is the world's sole supplier of this aromatic wood and oil.

Sandalwood oil, which is extracted from the wood by distillation, is used in perfumes, soaps, shampoos, and other beauty aids. It has a soft, smooth fragrance with a slight hint of rose. The *tika,* or dot that Hindu women place on their foreheads between the eyes, symbolizing "the gaze within," is made with sandalwood paste.

The word "sandalwood" comes from the Sanskrit *chandana.* The oil is found only in the heartwood of the tree and takes thirty years to form. To get to the heartwood, loggers leave sandalwood logs to termites, which slowly eat through the sapwood but cannot injure the hard inner core. The dense, fine grain of sandalwood's scented heartwood has made it the preferred wood for carving jewel boxes, reliquaries, beads, and statues. The sawdust that results from these carvings is made into a paste with gum arabic, a binder with no scent of its own, and is fashioned into *agarbhattis,* or incense sticks.

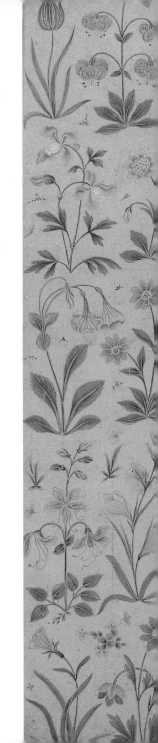

The scent of flowers and other plants was so central to Indian culture that few decorative arts—from ceremonial weapons to wall tiles—were left free of floral embellishment. This 5¹/₂-inch (14 cm) perfume bottle, mold-blown in the second half of the 18th century, is enameled and gilded with a scene of a young couple surrounded by the perfumed setting of a flowering garden. In Indian literature, gardens are familiar sites of romantic trysts.

Rogers Fund, 1921   21.26.11

Many Mughal albums filled with paintings and poetry are almost fragrant with the depictions of flowers. Most of India's flowering plants have been delicately and realistically portrayed on the borders of pages. In the example at right, lilies, tulips, and columbine are included in a border detail from an album assembled for Emperor Shah Jahan in the mid–17th century.

Purchase, Rogers Fund and The Kevorkian Foundation Gift, 1955   55.121.10.11

Patchouli is another aromatic that was long used in Indian culture before becoming a key item in modern perfumery. It is a tropical member of the mint family, and its name comes from an Indian word for "green leaf."

Still another Indian aromatic is vetiver (*Vetiveria zizanoides*), a member of the grass family. It has a strong, green smell that is so clean, dry, crisp, and almost harsh that the Indians say it dissipates heat and humidity. The fine roots of this plant were woven into fans and screens that were placed over the openings of a veranda and dampened with water. As the breeze passed through the screens and entered the interior of the palace or temple, it was perfumed and cooled. Today, vetiver's astringent quality makes it popular in men's colognes.

Champac is a member of the magnolia family, but it has an even sweeter scent. Champac and other scented flowers are made into garlands that are placed around the necks of rulers, statues of deities, and brides and grooms. During the Tang dynasty (618–905), Buddhist monks carried champac to China, where it became a popular shrub in the gardens of central and southern areas. With the solvent extraction process, this ancient favorite has become available to modern perfumery. The note is intensely floral, with fruit notes reminiscent of ylang-ylang.

The valley of Kashmir was the original home of the jasmine plant (*Jasminum* species), and India possesses an astonishing forty-three species of jasmine. Like champac, jasmine is woven into garlands for *puja,* or devotional acts, and the garlands are placed around the necks of both statues and officiants. In modern perfumery, this plant is known as the king of the flowers because it combines splendidly with almost any other scent. Arpège and Chanel No. 5 are perfumes rich in jasmine; Guerlain's Samsara is a true Indian blend of sandalwood and jasmine.

Cloves (*Syzygium aromaticum*), mentioned by the Sanskrit lexicographer Amarashimha in the sixth century, probably originated in the Moluccas, a group of islands in the East Indies. The leaves of the plant contain essential oil, but it is the bud that has the scent recognized today. Dried clove buds were exported from the East Indies to Europe via the Arab trade network and became indispensable in Renaissance sachets and pomanders. Just as they were in antiquity, the buds must still be picked laboriously by hand. The warm notes of clove are still a part of such men's colognes as Old Spice and such oriental-type women's fragrances as Tabu, Youth Dew, and Opium.

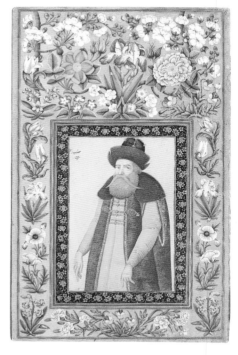

The Russian ambassador portrayed on this page from a 17th-century or early-18th-century Indian album is crowned and surrounded by an enormous variety of India's flowering plants. These include carnations, hyacinths, irises, poppies, primroses, several varieties of roses, tulips, violas and violets, and branches of a flowering tree. The page measures only 13 1/8 inches (33.3 cm) tall; thus, the flowers are minute and thoroughly astonishing in their fine detail.
Theodore M. Davis Collection, Bequest of Theodore M. Davis, 1915   30.95.174.4

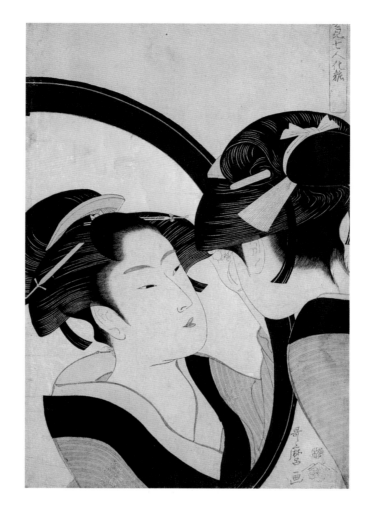

Scent in East Asia

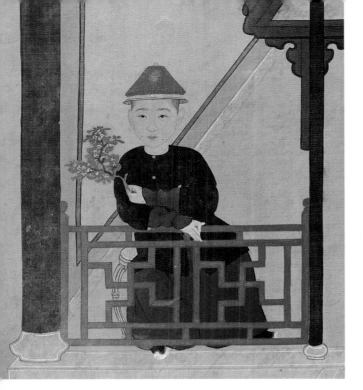

This young man in a detail from an early Qing dynasty painting (ca. 1662–1723) is holding a sprig of cassia, or osmanthus, a flower with an intense, sweet odor that is native to China. It appears in perfumery today as a costly floral absolute.

Anonymous Gift, 1952 52.209.3 D

On the previous page is *Beauty Admiring Herself in a Mirror,* by Kitagawa Utamaro (1753–1806), from the series of woodblock prints *Seven Beauties at Their Mirrors.*

Harris Brisbane Dick Fund, 1946 JP 3018

PERFUMES OF CHINA

Compared with the wealth of materials found in India, China's botanical contribution to perfumery was modest, which is not to say that it had no native aromatics. It did. Its flowering trees, such as camphor, cassia, citrus, peach, and apricot, have played an important part in perfumery. But China's key contribution to the story of perfume was the great boost it gave to trade.

China was barricaded from the Near East and the Mediterranean by the highest mountains on earth to the west and by impenetrable jungles to the south. However, the Silk Route wound its way north of the Himalayas, and from the ninth century—when Muslim traders first reached China's ports—through the fifteenth century, there was a brisk trade in aromatics. China not only had an enormous, prosperous population but also had a culture that valued pleasant scents. Thus, the Chinese were avid consumers of whatever fragrances were brought to their doors.

Among China's early trade gifts to the world were flowering fruit trees. The pear blossoms below are a detail from a scroll by Qian Xuan, painted in ink and color on paper in the Yuan dynasty, about 1235–1300.

Purchase, The Dillon Fund Gift, 1977.79
Photograph by Malcolm Varon

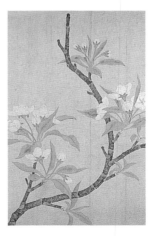

Trade made a variety of aromatics available to the Chinese and generated a lively home market for fine products for daily use, including incense burners. Many incense burners were modeled after shapes common to contemporary porcelains. As if to counter their austere designs, some bronze vessels, such as the example at right, were splashed with gilding. This incense burner was made in the late 16th or early 17th century, during the Ming dynasty.

H. O. Havemeyer Collection, Bequest of Mrs. H. O. Havemeyer, 1929   29.100.550

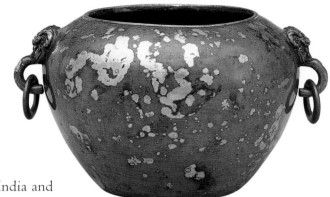

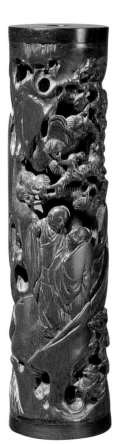

Trade goods traveled to and from India and the Arabian peninsula by land and sea. China exported its flowering trees, such as citrus, which reached the Mediterranean world in the late Middle Ages (and later traveled from there to Florida). In return, it received tropical hardwoods for making furniture, as well as sandalwood and aloeswood for incense. China also imported frankincense and myrrh, which were used in medicine, in cooking, and in sachets worn on the person. The appetite for these imports was so great that in the thirteenth century the Chinese government began to suffer a serious imbalance of trade.

"There was little clear-cut distinction among drugs, spices, perfumes, and incenses—that is, among substances which nourish the body and those which nourish the spirit," wrote sinologist Edward Schaefer of the Tang dynasty

Burning incense was a fashionable pastime among scholars and merchants during the late 16th and early 17th centuries, when this Ming-dynasty bamboo stand was made. It was carved by Zhu Sansong for holding stick incense: The openwork carving facilitated the release of fragrant smoke. The imagery depicts Laughter at Tiger Creek, a legendary story of the meeting of the Buddhist monk Huiyuan with the poet Tao Yuanming and the Daoist priest Lu Xiujing on Mount Lu.

Purchase, Friends of Asian Art Gifts, 1995   1995.271

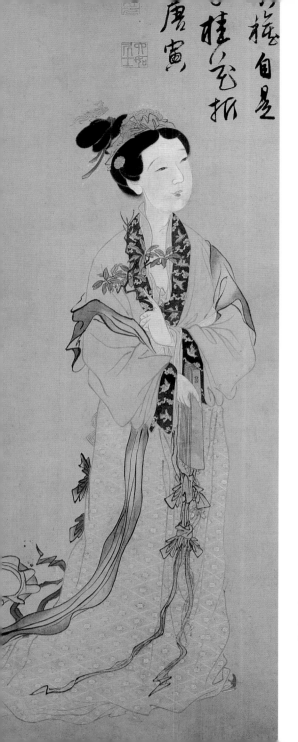

(618–906). "A man or woman of the upper classes lived in clouds of incense and mists of perfume. The body was perfumed, the bath was scented, the costume was hung with sachets. The home was sweet-smelling, and the office was fragrant, the temple was redolent of a thousand sweet-smelling balms and essences."

THE MANY USES OF SCENT

Women used many scented cosmetic oils that were based on sesame, rapeseed, or camellia oils. Sachets were worn in the folds of garments, and in the Tang dynasty a dance was performed that included the pelting of spectators with perfumed sachets. Rafters and storage chests were constructed of camphor wood, which lent its clean, astringent perfume to a room. Paneling for elegant buildings was made of *nanmu*, "southern wood," which has a cedarlike scent. Two aromatic trees called cassia were also enjoyed in various ways. One, a close relative of cinnamon, has aromatic bark that was ground into incense blends. The

The Chinese moon goddess Chang E is shown at left as painted by Tang Yin (1470–1524). She holds a branch of cassia, or osmanthus, and a fan in her hands. According to tradition, Chang E stole the elixir of immortality and resides in the moon. The artist links the goddess with the fragrant cassia flower in a poem:

> **She was long ago a resident of the Moon Palace,**
> **Where phoenixes and cranes gathered, and**
> **Embroidered banners fluttered in heavenly fragrance.**
> **Chang E, in love with the gifted scholar,**
> **Presents him with the topmost branch of the cassia tree.**

In Chinese, the characters for "cassia" and "nobility" are both pronounced *gui*. This painting in ink and color is a detail from a hanging scroll. Tang Yin was both an accomplished artist and poet.

Gift of Douglas Dillon, 1981   1981.4.2

This carved nephrite (jade) incense burner, dating from the late 18th or early 19th century, is part of an incense set that was made for use at home. It would have been accompanied by a matching vase for holding the spatula and tongs used for handling the incense, and a covered box for storing the imported aromatic. This vessel would have been lined with sand or ash to hold the burning incense. The style of this piece is typical of Chinese jades carved to resemble works produced at the Mughal courts of India. In the mid– to late 18th century, Mughal jade carvings were collected and studied by the Chinese emperor. He was particularly impressed by the thinness of the Indian pieces, and as a result, some late-18th-century works have thinner walls than were common in the Chinese tradition.

Gift of Herber R. Bishop, 1902   02.18.537 A-B

other, also known as osmanthus, was appreciated for its tiny white flowers, which have a rich, sweet scent. In modern perfumery, the first cassia is used as a blender in heavier perfumes, and the second as a floral absolute.

In the twelfth century, Zhan Shinan described placing orange blossoms in a burner and heating them until drops of liquid collected "like sweat." The drops were then poured over agarwood and kept in a sealed jar to produce a fragrance of "extraordinary elegance."

Of the "five precious things" placed on altars—two candleholders, two vases, and an incense burner—the burner always took pride of

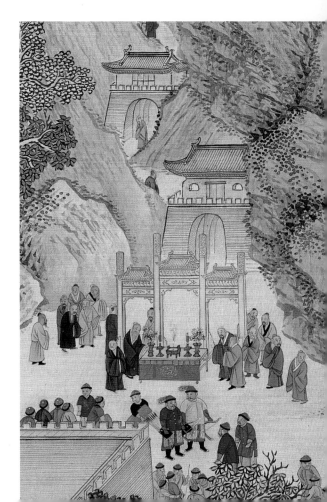

An incense burner is shown as central to the "five precious things" arranged on the altar in this detail from one of a series of twelve scrolls. The series, painted by Wang Hui (1632–1717) and his assistants, took three years to complete and records the events that took place during the Kangxi emperor's seventy-one-day southern inspection tour.

Purchase, The Dillon Fund Gift, 1979   1979.5

place in the middle. Clothes were perfumed by placing incense on special braziers. Camphor and juniper-seed oil were used in making ink so that when an ink stick was wetted for use, the scent was released. Scholarly men and women in China enjoyed the relationship between scent, form, texture, and color in the materials that made up the decor on or near the desk.

IN A CHINESE GARDEN

On a larger scale, Chinese scholars built themselves garden environments for the pleasure of all five senses: Trees, bushes, and other flowering plants were selected for beauty and fragrance alike. A typical scholar's garden of the Ming dynasty included tall pines, fragrant camphor trees, pavilions built of wood from the *nanmu* tree, and pools and channels of flowing water filled with the Asian lotus. A variety of citrus trees, which have scented blossoms, lined the meandering paths, as did wintersweet, which has jasminelike flowers that bloom in late winter. In fall, there was the crisp scent of chrysanthemums and the sweet perfume of osmanthus.

The pleasure of using incense sparked the production of fine decorative arts of every variety. The incense box above, made in the 14th century, is fashioned from carved and lacquered wood.

H. O. Havemeyer Collection, Bequest of Mrs. H. O. Havemeyer, 1929   29.100.713

Early spring brought the Chinese plum, which has great symbolism for the Chinese. It represents the triumph of life over adversity because the sweet flowers bloom in profusion on the naked boughs even before the foliage appears. Another icon of renewed hope was an orchid, the Chinese cymbidium, which Confucius himself praised for its wonderful perfume—elegant and never overbearing—so like the ideal personality.

Late spring brought the splendor of two peonies to the scholar's garden: the tree peony and the herbaceous peony, with their pink to deep red hues and floral-fruity scents. In the heat of summer bloomed the lotus (*Nelumbo nucifera*), whose huge flowers exude a musk-rose scent with hints of anise. The Confucian Zhou Dunyi described the lotus this way: "How untarnished it rises from its bed of mud, how modestly it bathes in the clear pond! It does not spread nor branch out. Its perfume is the purer the further it is away. It stands upright, gracefully. It is best to enjoy at a little distance."

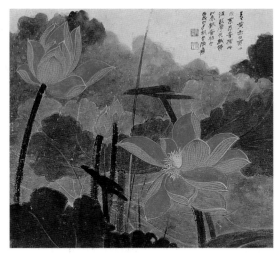

This image of lotuses, a detail from a hanging scroll, was painted by Zhang Daqian in 1946. The scent of lotus is both sweet and fruity. Buddhism adopted the flower as a symbol of its dharma, because although the roots of the lotus are buried deep in the mire, its flower is pure and its color is clear when it blooms above the waters.

Gift of Robert Hatfield Ellsworth, in memory of La Ferne Hatfield Ellsworth, 1986   1986.267.360

TECHNOLOGY AND PERFUMERY

From the tenth to nineteenth centuries, China was technologically advanced compared to much of the rest of the world. Several products and processes that originated in China in this period are still used in the contemporary perfume industry. Porcelain was developed in China in the seventh or eighth century and was brought to perfection during the Song dynasty (960–1276). Fine porcelain with a glasslike glaze makes wonderful containers for perfumes because it is as nonporous and nonreactive as glass.

The Chinese also made a great improvement in distillation techniques. They introduced a step in the procedure by which ethyl alcohol is extracted from wine, cooling the condenser by means of cold water. This step would

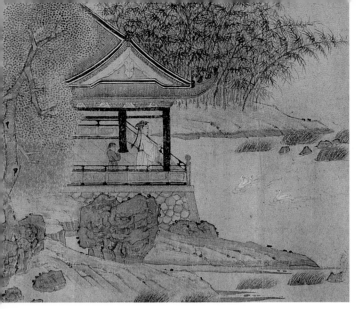

Filled with scented plants, the classical scholar's garden was the ideal place to visit when one's mind was in need of refreshing. The painting above records a moment during a literary event where China's greatest calligrapher, Wang Xizhi, wrote out his most famous calligraphic work. This detail of a handscroll by Qian Xuan (ca. 1235–1300) shows Wang Xizhi in a garden pavilion, gaining inspiration for his calligraphy by studying the graceful movements of geese.

Gift of The Dillon Fund, 1973   1973.120.6

eventually give Europeans of the early Renaissance insight into perfecting the distillation process, which led to the regular production of alcohol of high proof.

THE SCENTS OF JAPAN

The refinements of Chinese culture were carried to Korea and then across the East China Sea to Japan by monks and trade delegations, particularly during the Tang and Song dynasties. However, everything that the Japanese imported—calligraphy, painting, porcelain manufacture, papermaking, horticulture, and architecture—they also adapted and created anew. Thus, many of the Japanese uses of fragrance paralleled yet transformed those of China.

The Japanese burned incense in their temples and also created an incense-savoring ceremony, very much like the tea ceremony, in which the participants were given unlabeled samples to smell and match by scent alone. The enjoyment of incense has the name of *koh-do*, "the way of scent," which is akin to *cha-do*, "the way of tea." As had been done in China, the

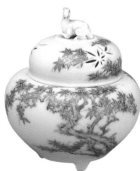

The Chinese enjoyment of incense was transferred to countries throughout East Asia. Japan adopted the practice of burning incense, making its own styles of burners for incense ceremonies. The underglazed-blue porcelain incense burner at left, only 3¹/₄ inches (8.3 cm) tall, has a tiny deer for a finial and leaf-shaped cuts for the smoke to escape. This type of porcelain, known as Hirado ware, was made at Mikawachi, near the famous porcelain-manufacturing city of Arita, beginning in the mid–17th century. Much Hirado ware of the 18th and 19th centuries was exported to Europe.

Gift of Charles Stewart Smith, 1893   93.3.11

In Japan, the materials used in making the accoutrements for incense were often quite precious. This incense box, made in 1876 by Ogawa Shomin, is decorated with *makie*, "sprinkled lacquer," and inlaid with mother-of-pearl flowers. The Japanese alone have specialized in producing *makie*, which is done by sprinkling powders of real gold and other precious metals over lacquered objects while they are still wet. The sprinkling of gold is done only by master artists.

Rogers Fund, 1936   36.100.165 A-B

Japanese made use of an incense clock. Because the stick incense that they fashioned out of aromatic sawdust and gum arabic was of a consistent quality, it was possible to calculate the time it would take to burn. The amount a client was charged for his time spent with a geisha was calculated by the number of incense tapers he went through—the scents of time.

OF JAPANESE ORIGIN

More unique to the Japanese are inro. These are diminutive lacquer cases, often designed as nesting tiers, that were hung on a clasp in the kimono by a silken cord. The wearer might store medicines, aromatics for

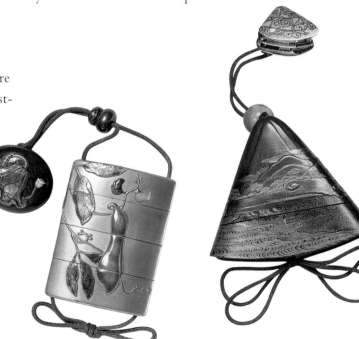

Inro, boxes for holding medicines and scents, are works of art unique to Japan. The two gold-lacquered examples at right were made in the 18th century.

Right: Inro signed by Mochizuki Hanzan
Rogers Fund, 1936   36.100.188
Photograph by Sheldan Collins

Far right: Inro signed by Kajikawa
Rogers Fund, 1913   13.67.93

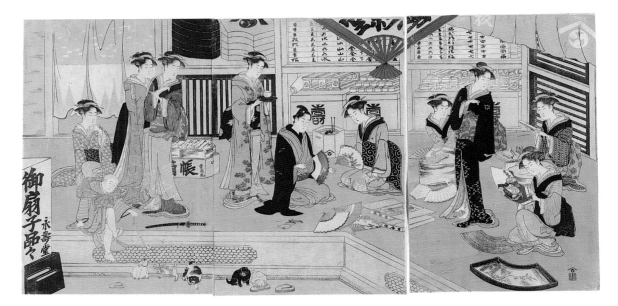

The folding fan, which could be used to waft soft scents as well as to cool the person, was invented in Japan. In about 1789, the artist Utagawa Toyokuni created this woodblock print triptych, which records a scene of women in a fan shop. The moment is clearly a social event. Beautifully dressed and coiffed women examine the artwork on fans, drink tea, and chat, while incense burns on a stove in the background.

The Howard Mansfield Collection, Purchase, Rogers Fund, 1936   JP 2725

inhaling, perfumes, or other small things in the inro's different sections. Exquisitely designed, the finest inro are precious works of art, decorated with carving or with imagery depicted in gold and silver powders. The modern perfume Opium is packaged in a container modeled on a red lacquer inro.

The Japanese enjoyed the use of scented oils and powders, hiding sachets among the folds in their kimonos. Among some of the other perfume-related products that originated in Japan are the *fusego*, a special rack for holding the kimono while it steeped in the smoke of incense, and the *kohmakura*, a headrest that emanated fragrance, which perfumed a court lady's hair while she slept. The Japanese also invented the folding fan, later made by the Chinese of sandalwood, which wafted its soft scent as it was used. Sandalwood fan manufacture is still an industry in the ancient Chinese city of Hangzhou.

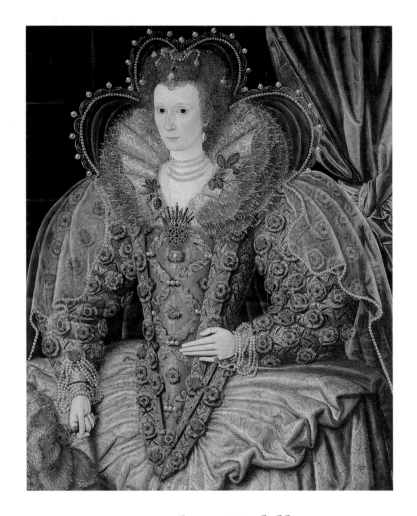

Scent in the Middle Ages
and the Renaissance

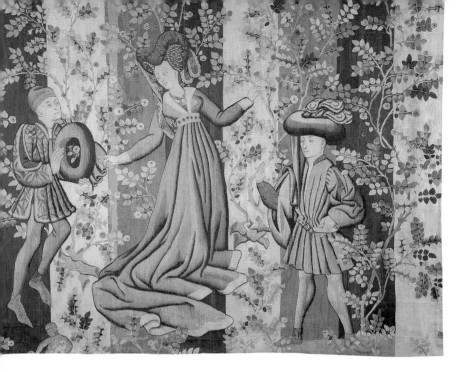

REAWAKENING TO SCENT

The story of Western perfumery ended for a time with the fall of Rome in the fifth century A.D. What was left of the craft was not perfumery directly, but the vestiges of medicine and pharmacy retained by monks in cloistered gardens during the sixth through eleventh centuries. The herbs they grew included clary sage, lavender, thyme, rosemary, and valerian. Most herbs were reserved for healing, for perfumery was nonexistent and ornamental horticulture was rudimentary.

Two early studies of herbs were *De Viribus Herbarum* (*On the Powers of Herbs*) by Odo of Meung, in France, in the early twelfth century, and *Causae et Curae* (*Causes and Cures*), by Abbess Hildegarde of Bingen (1098–1179), in Germany. She accorded high praise to lavender, a uniquely European scent with an uplifting herbal note.

Europeans in the Middle Ages were unfamiliar with most manufactured perfumes, but they did make use of scent. The lady and gentlemen in the tapestry fragment above conduct their meeting in a rose garden. The tapestry was made in the southern Netherlands about 1450–55.
Rogers Fund, 1909   09.137.2

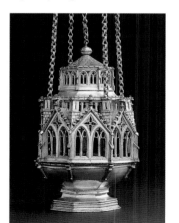

On the previous page is a portrait of a noblewoman by an unknown British painter of the late 16th century.
Gift of J. Pierpont Morgan, 1911   11.149.1

Throughout Europe in the Middle Ages and the Renaissance, the scent of incense was familiar to many through its use in churches. This silver censer, designed to look like a Gothic building, was swung from chains as the smoke emerged through the openwork windows. It was made in the Rhineland in the early 15th century and was used at the cathedral of Basel, in Switzerland.
Gift of J. Pierpont Morgan, 1917   17.190.360

Europe's first medical school opened in 1220 at Montpellier in Provence, France, where the chalky soil and warm climate are perfect for cultivating many aromatic plants. In centuries to come, Montpellier would rival the nearby town of Grasse as the center of perfumery, and the fields around the two towns would be redolent with the scent of herbs and flowers such as lavender, carnations, violets, jasmine, and roses.

THE DISCOVERY OF ALCOHOL

Chemists had continued to try their hands at distilling plant products ever since the process was discovered in Alexandria in the second century A.D. In 1320, Italian workers finally perfected the craft. They found that by insulating their equipment very well and cooling the tube that led vapors off the boiling distillation pot, they were able to produce a result

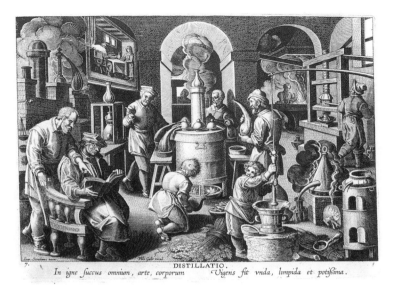

Distillation is the title of the image above, engraved by Philipp Galle in the 16th century, after a design by Jan van der Straet. The scene celebrates science and technology. A still billows steam, a man presses liquid with a screw-turned vise, a boy crushes herbs with a countersprung pestle, and a philosopher—wearing newly invented spectacles—reads a book of recipes. Harris Brisbane Dick Fund, 1934 34.30.8

Little dragons appear to be clinging to either side of the neck of this pear-shaped rosewater caster. The polished screw top is perforated so that the perfume can be sprinkled out. Made in London in about 1580, the caster stands 4³/₄ inches (12.1 cm) tall. It may have originally been fashioned as a bottle to hang from a cord, with the foot and perforated top added later. Gift of Irwin Untermyer, 1968 68.141.154

that was close to ninety-five percent alcohol. The first distillery in Europe was set up in the city of Modena, Italy. People at that time were so in awe of the new water look-alike with its burning taste that they called it *aqua mirabilis,* "marvelous water," and *aqua vitae,* "water of life." The first true perfumes—tinctures of essential oil in alcohol—were known as waters, too. (Today, true perfume is twenty-two to thirty percent essential oil and the rest alcohol, with some water.)

THE FIRST NAMED PERFUMES

In about 1370, fifty years after the discovery of alcohol, Queen Elizabeth of Hungary inspired the first named perfume, Hungary Water, an alcohol-based extract of rosemary and lavender. According to legend, the hermit who blended and presented the fragrance to the queen assured her that it would preserve her great beauty unimpaired until death. It seems to have worked, for at the age of seventy-two, Elizabeth of Hungary married the king of Poland.

In 1379, another named perfume, Eau de Carmes (Water of the Carmelites), was compounded of angelica, melissa, and other herbal oils by the Carmelite nuns of the abbey of St. Juste in France. A third early perfume was simply titled "Lavender Water." For a long time, alcohol-based perfumes were drunk as breath fresheners, although today perfumers are required by law to add a bitter substance such as quassia to the alcohol or to denature it to make it unfit for drinking.

Albarellos, or apothecary jars, were used throughout the Renaissance to store herbs and medicine. Although some had ceramic tops, most were sealed with caps of tightly fitting parchment or muslin. This *albarello,* made in Valencia, Spain, in the 15th century, has a luster glaze meant to simulate the sheen of precious metals.
The Cloisters Collection, 1956 56.171.91
Photograph by Schecter Lee

During the Renaissance, the Italian nobility enjoyed a vogue for regular bathing. The influence may have come from Italy's extensive trade with Islamic and Asian countries. The bathing process might have looked somewhat similar to the depiction in Giuseppe Chiari's *Bathsheba at Her Bath*, right, painted in about 1700.
Gift of Mario Modestini, 1993   1993.401

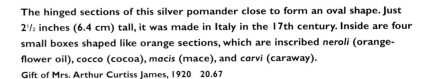

Further investigation into distilling continued, and by 1500 essential oils had been successfully extracted from pine, frankincense, cedar, and sweet flag. During the next forty years, the list would swell to include agarwood, sandalwood, anise, juniper, cardamom, fennel, and nutmeg.

RENAISSANCE PLEASURES

With the Renaissance, Europe's zest for experimentation burgeoned. As trade with the East expanded and exotic goods appeared on the market, many European craftsmen were inspired to create new products themselves. Weavers produced fine fabrics for men's and women's fashions; ceramists created brilliantly glazed household wares in great variety; and silversmiths and goldsmiths perfected their arts. Some of their products

The hinged sections of this silver pomander close to form an oval shape. Just 2¹/₂ inches (6.4 cm) tall, it was made in Italy in the 17th century. Inside are four small boxes shaped like orange sections, which are inscribed *neroli* (orange-flower oil), *cocco* (cocoa), *macis* (mace), and *carvi* (caraway).
Gift of Mrs. Arthur Curtiss James, 1920   20.67

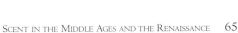

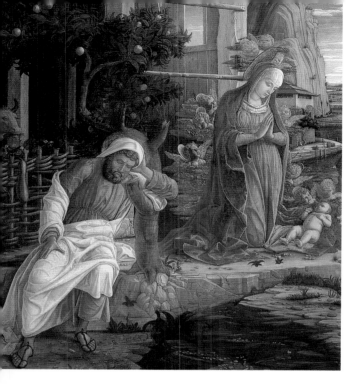

Oranges, which are native to China, were new to Europe in the late Middle Ages. Andrea Mantegna was clearly aware of orange trees and their beautiful golden fruit when he painted *The Adoration of the Shepherds*, a detail of which is shown at left. The work seems to have been painted for Borso d'Este, the ruler of Ferrara, and dates to about 1451.

Purchase, Anonymous Gift, 1932 32.130.2

would appear on the dressing table in the form of vials, jars, and cosmetic boxes. Information regarding science and health also flowed in from the East and sparked a renewed interest in hygiene. Members of the Italian upper classes fell into the habit of relaxing in the bath and washing their hair once a week.

Because the city of Venice was the European leader in trade for much of the Middle Ages and the early Renaissance, it was also the first place where imported goods and newly refined tastes appeared. One observer of the period noted that in Venice "everything was scented, gloves, shoes, stockings, shirts, and even coins. As if this were not enough, people kept objects made of scented pastes on their persons and held ambergris crowns in their hands."

From the Middle Ages onward, England's upper classes were accustomed to rinsing their hands with rose water before a banquet. This silver-gilt rosewater ewer, which has a matching basin, was made in about 1610 for Henry Frederick, Prince of Wales, the eldest son of James I of England (James VI of Scotland). Royal silversmith Simon Owen worked the appropriate imagery of roses and dolphins in rippling waters into the design.

Gift of Irwin Untermyer, 1968 68.141.136
Photograph by Schecter Lee

Venice was not the only site where perfumes were of concern: The upper classes in every Italian city delighted in the pleasures of scent. The great Renaissance women Isabella d'Este, Caterina Sforza, and Isabella Cortese published their recipes for fragrances. Ladies carried or wore pierced silver globes filled with ambergris or musk. These globes were known as pomanders, a corruption of the French *pommes d'ambre*, literally "apples of ambergris."

Leonardo da Vinci performed experiments with infusions of flowers and herbs in alcohol, or *acquarzente*, at the court of Ludovico il Moro in Milan. He also attempted experiments with an enfleurage of orange blossoms in almonds so that the almond oil would have a floral scent.

The introduction of orange trees, jasmine plants, and rosebushes in Europe was also the result of Italy's trade with the East. Rose water became as popular in Italy as it had been in Persia. Italian diners washed their hands with it until the knife and fork came into general use in the late 17th century. Rose water and other perfumes were produced at many monasteries. In Florence, the pharmacy of the monastery of Santa Maria Novella provided the de' Medici family with all its floral and herbal essences.

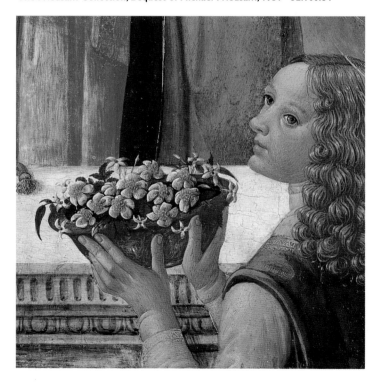

Sweetbriar and jasmine are offered in a basket in this detail of a 15th-century painting by Cosimo Rosselli, entitled *Madonna and Child with Angels*. Sweetbriar is native to Europe, but jasmine, now one of the most important plants in perfumery, was introduced into Italy during the Renaissance. When Italian customs were transposed to France in the 16th century, jasmine cultivation was brought as well. The Friedsam Collection, Bequest of Michael Friedsam, 1931   32.100.84

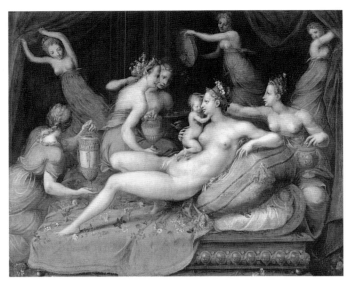

In classical mythology, the love affair between Venus and Mars resulted in the birth of Cupid. The Master of Flora painted this *Birth of Cupid* in the second half of the 16th century. Venus's bed is strewn with fragrant blossoms and herbs, including rosemary, pansies, pinks, and sweetbriar. All of these plants are native to Europe and were appreciated for their scents.
Rogers Fund, 1941   41.48

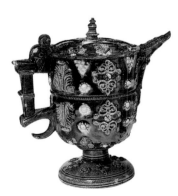

This earthenware rosewater ewer was made in Avignon, France, in the second half of the 17th century. Although working with a common clay, the potter who made this piece created a ewer fit for use on a fine table, through the use of embellished details and colorful lead glazes.
Gift of G. J. Demotte, 1923   23.201

NEW SCHOLARSHIP

The sixteenth century saw the publication of many volumes on plants, with descriptions of how to use them as medicines, perfumes, and cosmetics. The botanical woodcuts that accompany the text of Piero Andrea Mattioli's *Commentary* are so beautifully rendered that they continue to be popular as illustrations. In 1555, Giovanni Roseto published his illustrious *Secrets of the Art of Perfumery*, "for the enrichment of body and soul." And in *Magia Naturalis*, Giovanni Battista della Porta (1536–1615) advocated the use of glassware when extracting essential oils and alcohol from plants because it was nonreactive. Fortunately at that time, the Venetians were perfecting the art of glassmaking on the island of Murano.

In the fifteenth century, the French did not completely lack knowledge of scent. Well-heeled ladies and gentlemen wore small sachets, or *coussines*, in their clothing and had molded-clay bottles, called *oyselets de chypre*, for their perfume. But in large part, French perfumery skills of the period lagged far behind those of Italy. It would not be until the early sixteenth century, during the reign of Francis I, that Italian tastes in matters of the arts, fashion, gardening,

These amber- and blue-glass perfume flacons were made in Orléans, France, sometime between 1690 and 1710. They were formed by blowing molten glass into a hearts-and-flowers mold and are fitted with pewter screw tops. It was easier to create brilliantly colored glass at that time than it was to achieve perfect clarity. France's glass industry would blossom under Louis XV in the 18th century.
Gift of Henry G. Marquand, 1883   83.7.22, 83.7.165

and architecture began to filter into France and to have a major impact on its customs.

Perfume Comes to France

In 1533, Francis I's son Henri II married the Florentine noblewoman Caterina de' Medici. This was an event that would lead to startling changes in French culture, for Caterina brought all the arts and refinements of Renaissance Italy with her. Caterina's perfumer, Renato Bianco, joined her in Paris and set up a shop on the Pont au Change; her alchemist, Cosimo Ruggiero, made the trip to France as well. With their arrival, France received its first lesson in the art of perfumery. In the next century, French interest in scent would outstrip that of the rest of the world. The area of Grasse, in the south of France, chosen by Caterina to produce fragrant harvests of perfumery herbs and flowers, is the mecca of perfumery today.

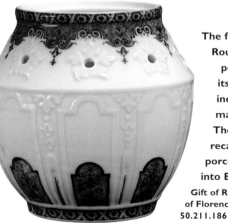

The factory of Louis Poterat, in Rouen, France, produced this potpourri jar (now missing its lid) in about 1690. Only 5 inches (12.7 cm) tall, it is made of soft-paste porcelain. The blue-painted decoration recalls the look of Chinese porcelain, which was imported into Europe in the 17th century.
Gift of R. Thornton Wilson, in memory of Florence Ellsworth Wilson, 1950
50.211.186

Not everyone readily adopted the new Italian ways, however. Henri IV (1553–1610), for instance, considered them foppish, and contemporaries said that the king "stank like carrion." (Interest in bathing remained negligible in France in the

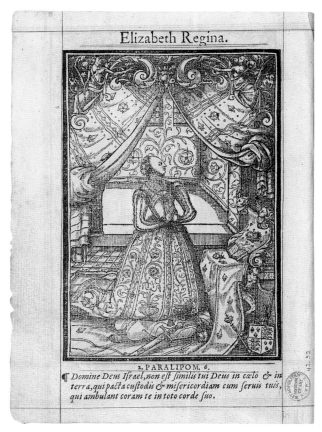

This dedication page from *A Booke of Christian Prayers*, or "Queen Elizabeth's prayer book," shows Elizabeth I at her devotions. Published in London by Richard Yardley and Peter Short in 1590, the volume was perfumed with musk. The scent can still be detected today.
Gift of Christian A. Zabriskie, 1942 42.32

sixteenth century.) Nevertheless, the movement toward better hygiene and care of the body slowly continued. Louis XIII (1601–1643) introduced the custom of wearing powdered wigs. His wife, Anne of Austria (who left some 340 pairs of scented gloves at her death), confessed to her contemporaries that she was very uncomfortable when it came to bad odors. She was told in turn that in recognition of her refined tastes, she would be carried off to hell in fresh linens and smelling of perfumes when she died.

Louis XIV (1638–1715) was supremely sensitive to odors. His perfumer, Monsieur Martial, was given the duty of composing a perfume for each day of the week. Under the adroit tutelage of Jean-Baptiste Colbert, Louis XIV's minister of finance, the south of France produced leather gloves perfumed with rose and orange blossoms, soap made from olive oil, and bottled scent.

The glovemaking industry was originally allied with perfumery in a single guild in France, but as the market for scent steadily increased, perfumery achieved independent guild status. In addition to the brisk business that Grasse and Montpellier did as purveyors of scented products to Louis XIV's court, they increasingly provided goods to customers outside of France's borders.

ENGLISH AROMATICS

During the late Middle Ages, England had a keen appetite for Eastern aromatics, brought to the port of Southhampton by Venetian traders. And in the sixteenth century under Elizabeth I, the country enjoyed a burst of interest in scent as the arts and pleasures of the Renaissance took hold. Sachets and silver pomanders were worn by Elizabethan ladies, as were necklaces strung with dried rose-buds that exuded their own perfume. Lavender, tarragon, marjoram, oregano, thyme, basil, mint, and other aromatic herbs and flowers of Europe made wonderful potpourris. Yet people found these scented blends far more interesting with the addition of Eastern spices such as clove, cinnamon, or cardamom.

This 5 3/8-inch (13.7 cm) silver spice box was made in London in 1602. Such boxes were introduced toward the end of the 16th century in response to the overseas trade in exotic spices. Once the trade routes were established, boxes with interior partitions containing sugar and spices became a favorite addition to the well-set table. Gift of Irwin Untermyer, 1968   68.141.277

Some Tudor manor houses had adjuncts of stillrooms, where the lady of the house might oversee the concoction of medicinal and fragrant extracts for "all and sundry purposes."

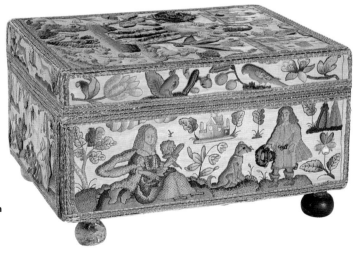

The Englishwoman who embroidered the panels for this dresser cabinet chose the subject of the five senses for her imagery. At left front, the sense of smell is represented by a lady holding a rose. Made between 1650 and 1675, the cabinet is 9 inches (22.9 cm) long. The white satin panels, stitched in petit-point and stump-work (which creates the three-dimensional details), are embellished with seed pearls and coral. Rogers Fund, 1929   29.23.1

The Queen's ladies and maids were accomplished in distilling cordials, medicines, and perfumes. And Elizabeth herself was known to visit the stillroom where her apothecary compounded "sweet waters." One Ralph Rabbards, "a gentleman studious and expert in Alchemical Artes," sent the queen a letter advertising his "waters of purest substance from odors, flowers, fruites, and herbes."

The scents of rose and animal musk were favored by the Elizabethans. Shakespeare often mentioned lavender, violet, marjoram, mint, civet, musk, and other scents in his writings, but he preferred rose above all. Ben Johnson wrote of the "casting glass," which was used to disperse scented waters in a room, like the *gulabdan,* of Persia: "His civet and his casting glass have helped him to a place among the rest."

Bucklesbury Street was the place where trade in herbs and scented products was concentrated in London—the very name conjured up cleanliness and pleasure. And when, in the early seventeenth century, England established the East India Company for trade with spice-growing regions of Asia, there was no longer a shortage of aromatics to choose from.

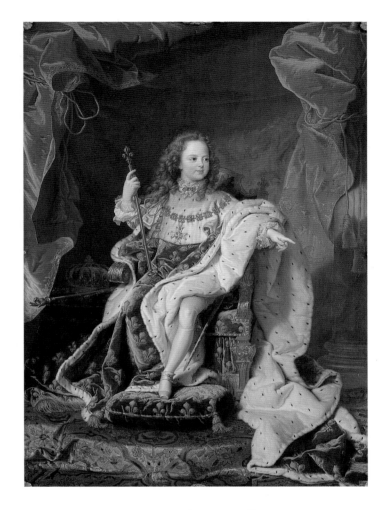

Scent in the
Eighteenth Century

◄►○◄►

The Perfumed Court

A fashion for pastel silks, powdered hair, panniered skirts, and beribboned bodices marked the Rococo style of dress in the eighteenth century. In France, the style was most intimately associated with Louis XV (1710–1774) and his mistress Madame de Pompadour (1721–1764). Above anyone else at midcentury, Madame de Pompadour established the standard of taste in fashion, beauty, and the arts.

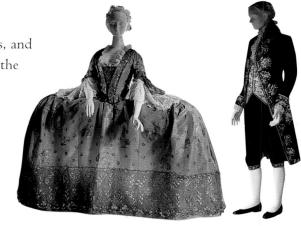

Jeanne Antoinette d'Etioles was the married daughter of a purveyor of army supplies when she first met the king at a ball and captured his interest. The king conferred a title on her, and d'Etioles became the Marquise de Pompadour. Elegant, intelligent, and accomplished, Madame de Pompadour was

The love of luxury was often refined to the point of artifice in Rococo fashion, as shown by this court gown from the mid–18th century. An elliptical hooped underskirt gives the silver-brocaded blue silk gown its 55-inch (139.7 cm) width. The making of fine men's clothing required a textile designer, fiber merchant, weaver, embroiderer, and tailor. This formal suit was made of patterned silk velvet in the last quarter of the 18th century.

Gown: Purchase, Irene Lewisohn Bequest, 1965 CI.65.13.1
Suit: Rogers Fund, 1932 32.35.12 A–C
Photographs by Sheldan Collins

Sculptor Jean Baptiste Pigalle was a favorite at the court of Louis XV. Pigalle's style expressed an honest naturalism. Between 1748 and 1751, Pigalle sculpted the marble bust of Madame de Pompadour at left, which does not flatter her, but does catch her humor, intelligence, and famously elegant neck.

The Jules Bache Collection, 1949 49.7.70

On the previous page is a painting by Hyacinthe Rigaud (1659–1743) of Louis XV at age five.

Purchase, Mary Wetmore Shively Bequest, in memory of her husband, Henry L. Shively, M.D., 1960 60.6

extremely influential within the court and beyond. She encouraged every phase of the decorative arts with her generous patronage, guided always by her excellent eye. The perfume producers of Grasse (and indeed all of Europe) owed much to her interest in fragrances. For the twenty years that Madame de Pompadour's life was linked to the king's, France's perfume business evolved from cottage craft to near industry, and Louis XV's court was dubbed *la cour parfumée*, "the perfumed court."

A PASSION FOR SCENT

In mid- to late-eighteenth-century France, ladies and gentlemen who followed fashion were scented from head to fingertip. The pearl-gray coiffures of the day got their color from powdered orrisroot, which comes from the rootstock of irises and has the odor of violets. Gloves were perfumed with neroli, distilled from the blossoms of the bitter orange. The most famous glove producer of the period was the family of Fargeon of Montpellier. Scented gloves remained a major fragrance product until the 1760s, when the French

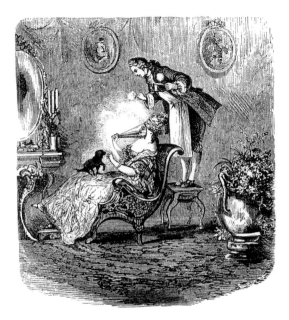

The fashion for powdering hair began toward the end of the 16th century and lasted about two hundred years. Hairstyles grew increasingly elaborate as the century went on. Sometimes poufs and other attachments of false hair were added to a person's own. As shown in the engraving above, powdering required the help of an assistant.

From *The Book of Perfumes*, by Eugene Rimmel, London, 1865. The Metropolitan Museum of Art, Thomas J. Watson Library

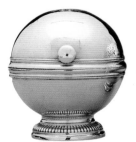
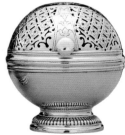

Soap and a sponge were stored in this pair of spherical silver boxes, made in France in about 1739, possibly by silversmith C. L. Gérard. Concocted and first used in Persia, soap was later introduced in Europe as a blend of olive oil and aromatics molded into balls.

Bequest of Catherine D. Wentworth, 1948   48.187.142, 143

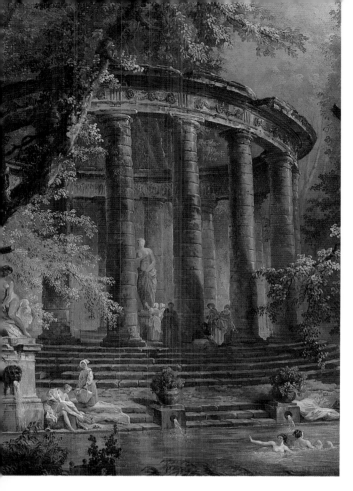

Madame de Pompadour helped to make bathing popular. In the detail of *The Bathing Pool* above, by Hubert Robert, the activity seems positively glamorous. The canvas was one of six commissioned for a boudoir in the Château de Bagatelle, near Paris, in the mid–18th century. Bathtubs at that date were made of marble, copper, or, less expensively, tin. Some had carved and upholstered arms and backs such as those on a fine chair or daybed.

Gift of J. Pierpont Morgan, 1917   17.190.29

government initiated a series of efforts to raise revenues by taxing hides. The city of Montpellier had invested so deeply in this one product that it went under completely, and the neighboring city of Grasse became the sole supplier to the perfume trade.

Madame de Pompadour was a strong advocate of frequent bathing. For those among the French upper classes less scrupulous in their hygiene, perfume was expected to cover a multitude of problems.

As bathing slowly became more commonplace, scented vinegars were used to tone the skin, and soaps were perfumed with lavender and other flowers with a clean herbal character. Like many ladies of the court, Madame de Pompadour spent hours on her toilette: To protect her beautiful complexion, she applied a scented astringent twice a week.

Pomades for the hair were also scented. They were made with an enfleurage of jasmine, violet, carnation, or hyacinth, or by macerating orange blossoms in hot fat.

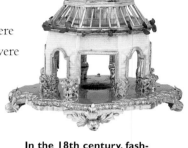

In the 18th century, fashionable people in France often added fragrance to their salons by means of a perfume burner. The example above, shaped like a tiny house, is one of a pair created in about 1750 from an earlier Chinese *blanc-de-chine* porcelain censer and French gilt-bronze mounts.

Bequest of George Blumenthal, 1941
41.190.64 A–B

To further enjoy the pleasures of scent, Madame de Pompadour spent thousands of francs on porcelain flowers that she sprinkled with perfume, and she always kept a blooming hyacinth bulb in a vase by her side. Incense burners and porcelain jars of potpourri were familiar features in the "intimate apartments" that Louis XV had made out of some of the larger salons at Versailles and the Petite Trianon. France's increasing trade with the Near East and India gave potpourri a richer blend of spices than was ever before possible. The rose was the central element of such blends, reinforced with lavender, clove, nutmeg, silvery wisps of oakmoss, and powdered orrisroot.

THE ORIGINS OF EAU DE COLOGNE

The most celebrated blended scent of the age, eau de cologne had its origins in Italy and Germany, but its reputation was made with its complete adoption by the French nobility. The scent's history begins with an Italian barber, Gian Paolo Feminis, born in Val Vigezzo, near Milan, who left his homeland to seek his fortune in Germany. In 1709 he began marketing Aqua Admirabilis, a distilled "water" based on a refined grape spirit. It was scented with herbs and flowers that were part of the Italian perfumery tradition: neroli, bergamot, lavender, and rosemary.

The product was very well received by customers in Cologne, and Feminis soon summoned another member of his family north to help in the business.

Porcelain potpourri containers of the 18th century came in many shapes and sizes. The example at right, made at the Sèvres porcelain factory in about 1763, is one of a pair of potpourri vases modeled as towers with projecting cannon muzzles. The walls are painted with trophies of war and laurel wreaths, both symbols of victory. The vase stands 22¹/₂ inches (57.2 cm) tall on its gilt-bronze mount.

Gift of R. Thornton Wilson, in memory of Florence Ellsworth Wilson, 1956   56.80.1

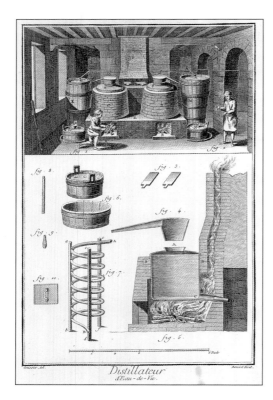

Distillateur
d'Eau-de-Vie.

French philosopher and dramatist Denis Diderot (1713–1784) was the editor of a multivolume encyclopedia that was published between 1759 and 1771. It examined and depicted craftsmen at their work in virtually every art and trade in France, including that of distillery. The top section of the engraving at left depicts a distillery worker stoking the fire under a large still. The lower section shows the various part of a still, illustrating how the process of distilling works.

Harris Brisbane Dick Fund, 1933 33.23

Giovanni Maria Farina (1685–1766) joined his uncle in Cologne, put the successful formula into writing, and in 1732 took charge of the business. As the business expanded, so did the number of would-be Farinas in the city. Many other perfumers opened shop, each claiming to be a descendant of the Farina family, each claiming to have the true formula. French troops stationed in Cologne during the Seven Years' War brought this wonderful "water" back to France, where it was dubbed "eau de cologne." The scent was particularly irresistible to Madame de Pompadour's successor, Madame Du Barry, who bought great quantities of it.

The French took their perfume seriously in the 18th century. This pocket-sized scent bottle, made in Paris between 1762 and 1768, is made of gold worked with chasing in a feathery design. A gold chain prevents the stopper from getting lost.

Bequest of Catherine D. Wentworth, 1948 48.187.482

FAVORITE FLOWERS

Notwithstanding the success of eau de cologne, most perfumes of the eighteenth century consisted of a single note, such as jasmine, neroli, or ambergris blended with alcohol. Traditional rose water and water of violets, for example, were favorites of Marie Antoinette. Millefleurs was one

French incense burners of the 18th century were known as *cassolettes* or *brûle parfums*. This one, made in about 1775, stands 40 inches tall (101.6 cm) on its carved- and gilded-wood base. The top section at one time was fitted with a small stove or spirit lamp, called a *réchaud*, over which pastilles or sweet-smelling essences were heated. The Paris guild of *parfumeurs* produced the ingredients that released these delicious odors. The aromatic fumes escaped through the ornamental perforations on the lid.

Purchase, Gift of Mr. and Mrs. Charles Wrightsman, by exchange, 1983   1983.313 A-C

of the few perfumes that was compounded from the essential oils of several flowers in a bouquet or potpourri enfleurage. Perfumers had also begun experimenting with seed extracts, such as those of almond and apricot, carried in various oils.

Enfleurage techniques were improved in the eighteenth century, and a literature of the French perfume industry developed. *The Chemistry of Taste and Scent,* by Polycarpe Poncelet, appeared in 1755 and promised to instruct how to "compose fragrant waters with facility." M. Dejean published his *Treatise of Scents* in 1764. In 1774, Larbalestier Petit published the *New Chemistry of Taste and Scent,* which claimed to teach how to make perfumes "at little expense." About the same time, Denis Diderot completed his *Encyclopaedia,* which included engravings of the distilling process. It was of service to both the French fragrance and distilled-spirits industries.

Until the early 1700s no one in Europe could make true porcelain. It required a particular white clay and a fusible white stone that could be fired at high temperatures, making it extremely hard. Even then, many factories continued to produce "soft-paste" porcelain, which was fired at lower temperatures. This soft-paste potpourri jar was produced in Chantilly, France, in about 1735.

The Jack and Belle Linsky Collection, 1982   1982.60.27 A-B

Known in their time as "toys," figural scent bottles such as these from Chelsea, England, were given as tokens of love and friendship in the 18th century. They were produced in an enormous variety of forms and sometimes bore affectionate inscriptions. Each of the figures in this group was made of soft-paste porcelain between about 1755 and 1765.

Gift of Irwin Untermyer, 1964   64.101.532 A–B, 568 A–B, 584 A–B, 593 A–B, 609 A–B

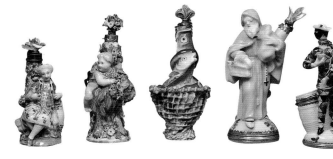

PORCELAIN IS INTRODUCED

The technical skills for designing and making new types of containers for holding scent developed with the fragrance industry. What made the use of potpourri so charming in the eighteenth century was the use of painted porcelain jars, which were set out on shelves and tabletops to hold aromatic floral blends. For years, European ceramists had been trying to reproduce imported Chinese porcelain, which, like glass, did not react with essential oils. In 1709, a German chemist working for the court at Meissen in Saxony was the first to reproduce porcelain successfully. Although attempts were made to keep the process secret, word got out, and as the eighteenth century progressed, factories in Vienna, Florence, and other European cities were producing high-quality, hand-decorated hard-paste porcelain. At the same time, many companies continued to manufacture soft-paste (or imitation) porcelain and other ceramics.

From the 1750s on, the factory at Chelsea, England, produced little perfume bottles shaped like harlequins, birds, animals, flow-

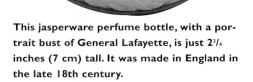

This jasperware perfume bottle, with a portrait bust of General Lafayette, is just 2³/₄ inches (7 cm) tall. It was made in England in the late 18th century.

Purchase, Joseph Pulitzer Bequest, 1942   42.76.12 A–B

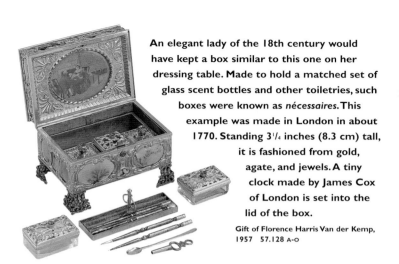

An elegant lady of the 18th century would have kept a box similar to this one on her dressing table. Made to hold a matched set of glass scent bottles and other toiletries, such boxes were known as *nécessaires*. This example was made in London in about 1770. Standing 3¼ inches (8.3 cm) tall, it is fashioned from gold, agate, and jewels. A tiny clock made by James Cox of London is set into the lid of the box.

Gift of Florence Harris Van der Kemp, 1957   57.128 A-O

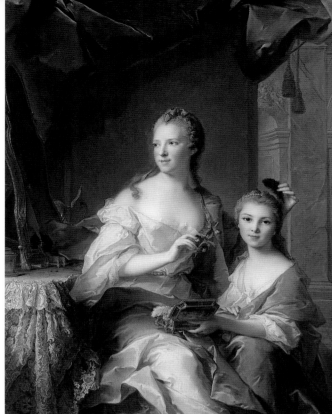

In the detail of Jean Marc Nattier's 1749 double portrait above, Madame Marsollier assists her young daughter at making her toilette. For fashionable French women in the 18th century, it was common to spend hours at the dressing table. Even very young women powdered their hair and rouged their cheeks. Magnificent bottles and boxes were made to hold their cosmetics and perfumes.

Bequest of Florence S. Schuette, 1945   45.172

ers, Chinese mandarins, and many other forms. In his Etruria, Staffordshire, factory Josiah Wedgwood manufactured pottery scent bottles of jasperware. France had no monopoly on perfume bottles during this period.

Glass production kept pace with the need for flacons. Although members of the nobility did not normally engage in any form of trade, eighteenth-century France—following the Venetian example—considered the making of glass an exception to this aristocratic rule.

The origins of the French glass company Pochet et du Courval go back to a royal grant in 1623, and the company still enjoys a brisk trade in perfume bottles today. The royal glass factory of Saint Gobain originated in 1665 with a grant from Louis XIV. This firm, too, continues to make bottles for the perfume trade. The Verrerie de Saint Louis, founded in 1767, was the predecessor to the Cristallerie de Baccarat, famous for its high-quality artistic glass. At first, bottles tended to be of a sea-green color, but French glassmakers' expertise in perfecting color and in blowing and molding glass burgeoned during the reign of Louis XV, leading to exquisite variety. Scent bottles were often created as tiny components of sets called *nécessaires,* which were luxuriously encased in tortoiseshell, leather, semi-precious stone, porcelain, enamel, or gold.

FAMOUS BRANDS ACROSS THE CHANNEL

Perfumery in Britain in the eighteenth century was a faint shadow of the industry developing across the English Channel in France. However, in 1708 Charles Lille (or Lilly) set up a shop in London and produced perfumes based on orange flower, musk, civet, and violet. In 1730, an emigrant from Minorca, Juan Floris, set up a wig and hairdressing business that expanded into perfumery. The company in his name, one of the oldest perfume houses in existence, still produces its traditional perfumes, scented powders, and potpourris. Thomas Yardley of London received his charter from George III in 1770 and brought out his famous lavender scent ten years later. It remains one of the world's most popular fragrances.

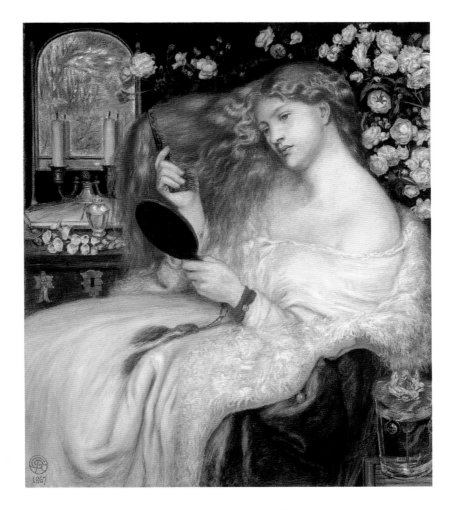

Scent in the
Nineteenth Century

⊳⊶⊷○⊶⊷⊲

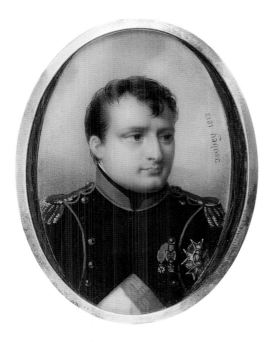

This miniature portrait of Napoléon I, only 2¼ inches (5.7 cm) tall, was painted on ivory by his court painter, Jean Baptiste Isabey, in 1812. Isabey was also responsible for designing many of Joséphine's gowns, which were made by Leroy, the most fashionable tailor of the day. Napoléon was known for his fastidious cleanliness during military campaigns, always traveling with his toiletries and bottles of cologne.

Gift of Helen O. Brice, 1942   42.53.5

On the previous page is Dante Gabriel Rossetti's 1867 painting of Lady Lilith at her dressing table.

Rogers Fund, 1908   08.162.1

NAPOLÉON AND JOSÉPHINE

France's perfume industry and all the other trades that catered to the aristocracy very nearly perished in the years after the French Revolution. Yet they were saved just in time. In 1804 Napoléon Bonaparte (1769–1821) crowned himself Napoléon I, emperor of France; his wife Joséphine (1763–1814) was made empress. A new era of elegance and extravagance began.

The powdered wigs and frock coats of the old regime were gone, but when Napoléon invited nobles who had fled during the war to return to the country, many of the cultivated graces of old France returned with them. Under Napoléon's orders, the silkweavers of Lyons, the glassmakers of Picardy and Normandy, the cabinetmakers of Paris, and the perfumers of Grasse resumed work. The decorative arts took on a classical look, befitting the republican ideals of the new government.

Business was good; for the first time, perfumers and other tradesmen were selling their products to a triumphant middle class, as well as to the aristocracy. Once again France was leading the world in the production of luxury goods. Napoléon also spurred economic progress by rewarding scientific talent and financing scientific research—including the study of essential oils and ethanol in the perfume industry.

FRENCH FASHION

Joséphine set the tone for the daring yet elegant "empire" look in clothing. She embodied a fashion evocative of Grecian maidens: narrow, high-waisted dresses with trains, tiny bodices, and revealing necklines. White was the preferred color for the new style of fine silk or gauzy cotton dress called the chemise. Bare shoulders in these light fashions were often warmed with Indian cashmere shawls. Napoléon himself had sent the first cashmere shawls to France during his Egyptian campaign. They would remain among the few imported textiles that he allowed to enter the country while he concentrated on boosting France's own textile industry.

When shipping their fine woolen shawls to Europe, Kashmiri weavers protected their products by layering the folds of cloth with the leaves and stems of dried patchouli, a tropical member of the mint family, which was an effective moth repellent. The warm, resinous scent of patchouli turned out to be as much of a draw for buyers in Paris as the colorful cashmere itself. After the scent was identified, it became popular in French perfumery. Patchouli is the fragrance to imagine wafting from the wrappings of women in the paintings of David, Ingres, Gérard, and Gros.

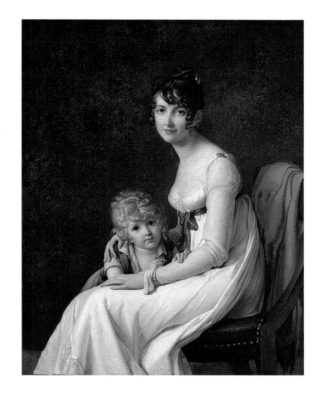

The double portrait above, of Madame Philippe Desbassayns de Richemont and her son Eugène, attributed to Marie-Guillelmine Benoist, was painted in 1803. Madame Desbassayns's filmy white dress epitomizes the Grecian-style fashions of the day.
Gift of Julia A. Berwind, 1953   53.61.4

This bottle was made in England in the mid–19th century. It is an unglazed porcelain known as Parian ware because it resembles Parian marble, which was used for classical sculpture.
Gift of Dr. Charles W. Green, 1947   47.90.97 A-B

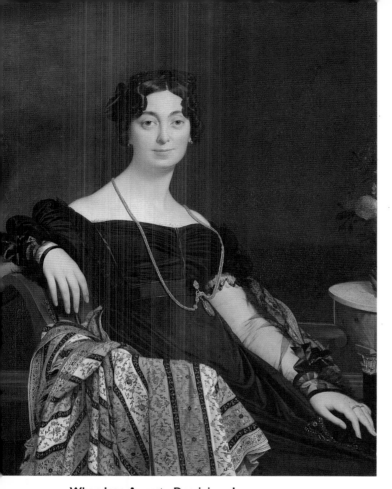

When Jean-Auguste-Dominique Ingres painted this portrait detail of Madame Jacques-Louis Leblanc in 1823, he included the preferred accessory of the day, the cashmere shawl. The aroma of patchouli that permeated Indian cashmere was new to Europeans in the 19th century, but it is a key scent in modern perfumery.

Catharine Lorillard Wolfe Collection, Wolfe Fund, 1918 19.77.2

Joséphine was fond of the scent of patchouli and also loved the perfume of rose. Her retreat at Malmaison was ringed by rose gardens that included every known species available. America's fashionable first lady Dolley Madison, who helped to make the high-waisted French dress style popular in the United States, was also partial to rose-scented colognes.

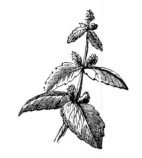

This illustration of patchouli is from *The Book of Perfumes,* by Eugene Rimmel, London, 1865.

The Metropolitan Museum of Art, Thomas J. Watson Library

Another of Joséphine's perfume passions was musk, a heavy, languorous scent that Napoléon could not abide. In 1810, when the emperor annulled their marriage in favor of his new consort, Marie-Louise, Joséphine took her revenge by saturating the imperial apartments in musk, which she knew was one of the most retentive of scents.

Elegance coupled with a certain republican restraint dictated the imperial style for men: slim fitted trousers, waist-length vests and jackets, high-collared shirts, and silk cravats. The emperor followed fashion very closely, but the new men's styles were also linked to the English dandy Beau Brummel in London. Napoléon was almost neurotically fastidious about cleanliness and good scent. He washed with the British soap Brown Windsor, made with bergamot, clove, and

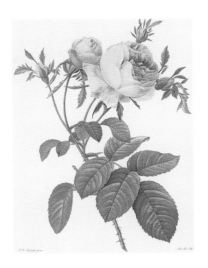

lavender oils, and he favored the scent of Farina's eau de cologne, often using several bottles a day. Led by Napoléon's example, the middle class in France and the rest of Europe developed a concern with cleanliness.

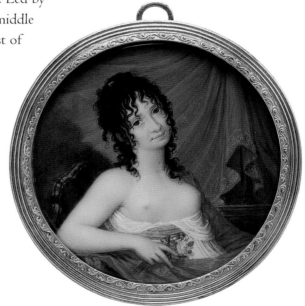

The perfume house of Antoine Chiris, founded in 1760, was one that managed to survive the Revolution, as did the ancient house of Tombarelly d'Escoffier. The former was among the first to start floral plantations in the soon-to-be established North African colonies: To this day, Morocco remains an important producer of fragrance materials. Other firms that weathered the political storms included Antoine Artaud, of Grasse, and J. F. Houbigant, which sold fragrance to the Bonapartes. The firm of François Lubin, which began under Napoléon and became linked with the name of his sister Princess Borghese, was the first to solicit the North American market, aiming particularly at the plantation culture of the southern United States.

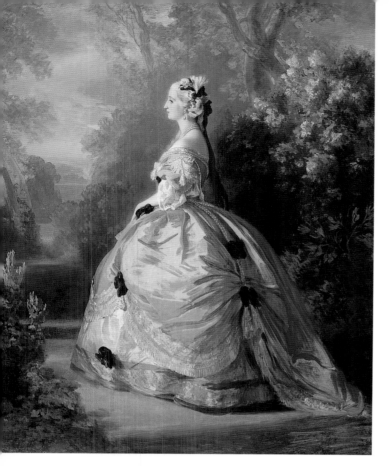

Franz Xaver Winterhalter painted this portrait of the empress Eugénie in 1854. Eugénie reintroduced good taste into French life. She patronized the fine crafts associated with the throne and saw to the creation of the Musée des Arts Décoratifs at the Louvre.

Purchase, Mr. and Mrs. Claus von Bülow Gift, 1978   1978.403

THE GLAMOUR OF EUGÉNIE

Fashion declined in the mid–nineteenth century, but it made a dramatic comeback with the empress Eugénie, consort of Napoléon III (Louis Napoléon, 1808–1873). Spanish-born Eugénie de Montijo de Guzman (1826–1920) created a rage for off-the-shoulder gowns and full-skirted crinolines—the perfect dresses for dancing the "naughty" new dance, the waltz. Eugénie's delight in ornamentation ensured the development of perfumery in France; in England, Queen Victoria was suppressing such trends.

Eugénie's sense of style was aided and abetted—and her gowns created—by the first of the great modern couturiers, the Englishman Charles Frederick Worth, who had emigrated to Paris to seek his fortune. Within ten years of Worth's arrival in Paris, only the empress herself could visit his shop without an appointment, and all new clients had to be recommended, like members of an exclusive club. In the 1920s, Worth's son Jean Phillip introduced the first Worth perfume, Dans la Nuit, as a free gift to clients, but its success proved that the perfume was a marketable entity of its own. The house of Worth has produced perfumes ever since.

For her scents, Eugénie patronized the house of Guerlain. It had originated as a shop on the Rue de Rivoli where Pierre François Guerlain sold his own fragranced soaps, scents, and smelling salts. (Smelling salts, a blend of fragrance and ammonia vapors, were required by ladies of the day because their tight corsets often

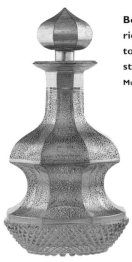

Bohemian glass, known for its brilliant color, fine cutwork, and engraving, was one of many European luxuries revived in the early 19th century. **By 1825, when this 8-inch (20.3 cm) perfume bottle was made, factories were producing large quantities of this immensely popular glass. This bottle's shape, onion-style stopper, and gilt-enamel decoration give it a Near Eastern look.**

Munsey Fund, 1927   27.185.352 A-B

provoked fainting spells.) In 1861 Guerlain created Eau Impériale for Eugénie. Like the original eau de cologne, Guerlain's was a light blend of citrus and lavender. The bottle was emblazoned with the bee symbol, the mark of the Bonapartes. Eau Impériale continues to be popular—one of the longest-lived of all fragrance creations.

Other new perfume houses that did a flourishing business in the encouraging climate of the 1860s included Frédéric Millot and the house of Molinard. The firm of Hermès, which was established in 1837, was heir to the long European tradition of scenting gloves. During this period, several important supply houses sprang up in Grasse to meet the

The bottle design for Eau Impériale, right, has changed very little since Eugénie's day.
Courtesy of Guerlain Inc.

The card at far right advertises the perfumes of Eugene Rimmel, who wrote the first comprehensive history of perfume in 1865.
The Jefferson R. Burdick Collection, Gift of Jefferson R. Burdick
Album 34

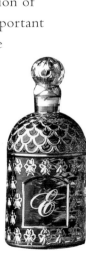

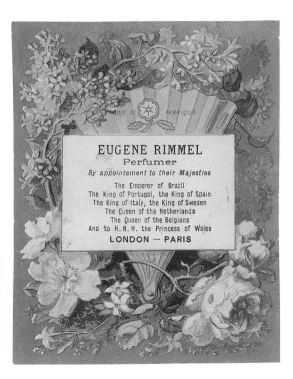

EUGENE RIMMEL
Perfumer
By appointement to their Majesties

The Emperor of Brazil
The King of Portugal, the King of Spain
The King of Italy, the King of Sweden
The Queen of the Netherlands
The Queen of the Belgians
And to H. R. H. the Princess of Wales
LONDON — PARIS

growing demand for essential oils: Roure Bertrand Dupont (now Givaudan Roure) and Robertet et Cie. are still in existence.

Fragrance Comes into Its Own

At the International Exhibition in Paris in 1867, perfumes and soaps were showcased in their own sections for the first time. In previous exhibitions they had appeared only marginally, as stepchildren of pharmacy and chemistry exhibits. Napoléon III helped to sever the link between fragrance and pharmacy by requiring the listing of all ingredients on pharmaceutical labels. Naturally, perfumers would rather be independent than divulge their secrets that way.

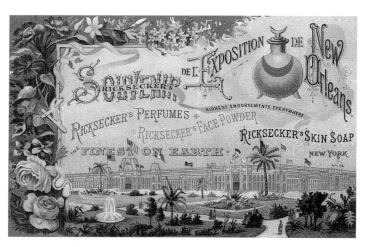

By the mid–19th century, national and international fairs and expositions featured displays of perfumes. At some, visitors could dip their handkerchiefs into perfume fountains. At other fairs, free samples of perfumes were distributed.

The Jefferson R. Burdick Collection, Gift of Jefferson R. Burdick   Album 34

Science and technology also brought perfumery a major step forward in the nineteenth century. Beginning in about 1835, discoveries that led to perfecting the process of solvent extraction enabled perfumers to use many flowers that had been unavailable to them before. Few flowers can withstand the rigors of distillation in boiling water. (Roses, orange blossoms, and ylang-ylang are among the exceptions.) By using chemical solvents, the manufacturers in Grasse were able to "dry-clean" the perfumes from such heat-sensitive flowers as jasmine, tuberose, honeysuckle, narcissus, mimosa, and Spanish broom. This process marked the start of modern perfumery.

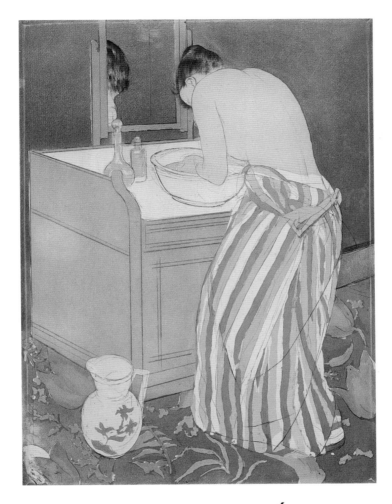

Scent in the Belle Époque
and the Jazz Age

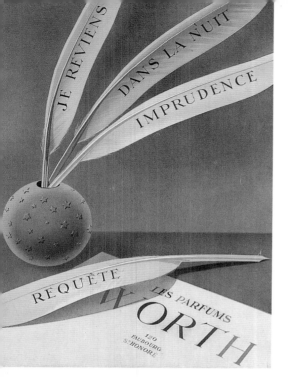

THE BELLE ÉPOQUE

Eugénie and Napoléon III's empire ended in 1871 with the disastrous Franco-Prussian War, but Paris eventually healed and the dazzling Belle Époque was ushered in. From the 1870s to the outbreak of World War I, the art of living was enjoyed by more people than ever before. The era witnessed the birth of flight and the arrival of the automobile, the telephone, the electric light, and the cinema. The Crystal Palace and the Eiffel Tower were erected in London and Paris. Travelers relaxed in grand style on luxurious transatlantic steamers. And France was the undisputed artistic capital of the world, where people could experience Rodin's sculpture, Monet's paintings, and the music of Debussy. In 1900 all of Paris turned out for the lavish Universal Exposition. Stylish women filled the cafés, dressed in the flowing fashions of Jacques Doucet and Charles Frederick Worth.

The house of Worth's first perfume was Dans la Nuit. It appeared in the 1920s in a frosted blue bottle covered with stars. As shown in the advertisement above, Worth went on to produce many other perfumes, including the immensely popular Je Reviens in 1932.

From *La Femme Chic*,
November–December 1945. The Metropolitan
Museum of Art, Irene Lewisohn Costume Reference
Library

On the previous page is Mary Cassatt's 1890–91 *Woman Bathing*, a dry-point, soft-ground etching and aquatint, fourth state, printed in color.

Gift of Paul J. Sachs, 1916 16.2.2

The Belle Époque also witnessed a veritable explosion in the luxury arts, including perfumery. The discovery of the process of solvent extraction in the 1830s had allowed perfumers to compose complex floral blends that had never before been

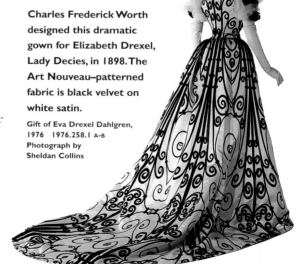

Charles Frederick Worth designed this dramatic gown for Elizabeth Drexel, Lady Decies, in 1898. The Art Nouveau–patterned fabric is black velvet on white satin.

Gift of Eva Drexel Dahlgren,
1976 1976.258.1 A-B
Photograph by
Sheldan Collins

possible. Still another important scientific breakthrough was yet to come.

SYNTHETIC SCENT

Through the development of organic chemistry, perfumers were also able to synthesize natural scents. In 1868, the English chemist William Perkin made coumarin, a synthetic that smelled like newly mown hay. Other synthetics followed: musk in 1888, vanilla in 1890, violet in 1893, camphor in 1896. The list continued to grow. In time, organic chemistry made it possible to reproduce the aroma of flowers whose natural scents cannot be obtained through any method of extraction, such as lilac, lily of the valley, and gardenia.

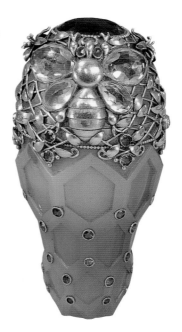

American designers did not lag behind their European counterparts in creating beautiful scent bottles. This 3⁵/₈-inch (9.2 cm) container was made by Tiffany and Company, of agate, gold, and semiprecious stones, in 1893.
Gift of the Duchesse de Mouchy, 1965   65.143

In the early twentieth century, European firms producing limited-edition art glass excelled in creating inspired designs for perfume. The example at left was designed by René Lalique, whose name is synonymous with beautiful glass. Only 3¹/₄ inches (8.3 cm) tall, the bottle is decorated in enamel with designs of capricorn beetles. Lalique also designed bottles for commercial perfumers. The company still produces elegant perfume bottles today.
Purchase, Edward C. Moore Jr. Gift, 1923 23.173.3

Among the great perfumes of the era was Fougère Royale, which had the soft green scent of ferns. It was created by Paul Parquet for Houbigant in 1882 and was the first perfume to make use of coumarin. The house of Guerlain produced Jicky as a family affair. It was created by Aimé Guerlain, who named it after young Jacques "Jicky" Guerlain. The perfume was sold in a bottle designed by Gabriel Guerlain, working with the glass makers of Baccarat. Jicky was a thoroughly modern scent that took advantage of both synthetics and the new absolutes—products of

Paul Poiret was the couturier of the moment when he created this silver lamé and green-silk fancy-dress costume in 1911. The revolutionary design—pants for women—was probably created for a garden party that Poiret held to publicize his oriental styles. Heralded as a Persian celebration, the party was called 1002 Nights. The three hundred guests were requested to wear Persian costume and were provided with appropriate costumes if they failed to show up wearing their own. The garden decorations included live monkeys and parrots in the trees.

Purchase, Irene Lewisohn Trust Gift, 1983   1983.8 A-B

solvent extraction. These components were backed up with orris, bergamot, and lavender oils. Although formulated for a male market, Jicky was taken up by the grandes dames of the period. In 1890 Aimé Guerlain brought out Cuir de Russie, and in 1895 the Guerlains created Le Jardin de Mon Curé, which was sold in a flacon by Baccarat. In creating Le Trèfle Incarnat for L. T. Piver in 1898, perfumer Jacques Rouché experimented with synthetics to achieve the perfume's soft, sweet-hay note.

THE REVOLUTIONARY POIRET

One of the great figures of the age and the most fashionable designer in Paris was Paul Poiret (1879–1943). Poiret initiated the concept of the couturier fragrance by creating Parfums Rosine, a company that produced fragrances as accessories for his fashions. This trend, the convergence of two French luxury arts—fashion and fragrance—turned out to be one of the most important in twentieth-century perfumery.

Poiret was Parisian to the core, the fact of which he never ceased to remind his rival Coco Chanel, who came from provincial Auvergne. An extremely vibrant and versatile

The sensuous lines of the French Art-Nouveau style in the early part of the 20th century are particularly appropriate for objects associated with beauty and the toilette. This hand mirror, made of cast bronze with a moonstone at the base of its handle, was designed by the noted sculptor Rupert Carabin in about 1907.

Gift of Rosenberg & Stiebel, Inc. 1979
1979.554

personality, Poiret helped to finance the careers of the artists Raoul Dufy, Sonia Delaunay, Erté, and Georges Lepape.

Poiret reveled in every art form. He loved Persian miniature paintings and mirrored them in his women's fashions with turbans, pantaloons, and dazzling colors. His ideal woman was elegant, luxurious, free of the constraints of the bustle and corset, and sheathed in fluid lines. The very names of Poiret's perfumes evoke the exotic image that he espoused: Le Fruit Défendu (Forbidden Fruit), Nuit de Chine (Chinese Night), Borgia, and Le Balcon (Balcony). His perfumer was the Spaniard Jean Alméras, who later created Joy for Jean Patou.

NEW SCENTS

In 1912 three important perfumes were introduced that are still with us. Houbigant's Quelques Fleurs, the first modern floral-bouquet perfume, was blended by Robert Bienaimé. Ernest Daltroff created Caron's Narcisse Noir using a special variety of the narcissus flower. And Guerlain produced L'Heure Bleue, blended with frankincense, labdanum, and balsam of Peru, along with several of the newest synthetics.

The houses of Houbigant, Caron, and Guerlain did not venture into couture but formulated and sold fragrances exclusively. In the early years of the century, the most celebrated newcomer to join the ranks of these perfume firms was François Coty (1876–1934), who was born Frances Sportuno, on the island of Corsica. (He took his

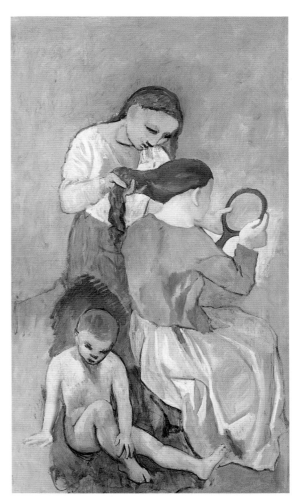

Picasso painted *La Coiffure*, above, in 1906. Although Picasso's art was, at times, radically new in style, its subject matter was often quite familiar.

Catharine Lorillard Wolfe Collection, Wolfe Fund, 1951, acquired from The Museum of Modern Art, Anonymous Gift   53.140.3

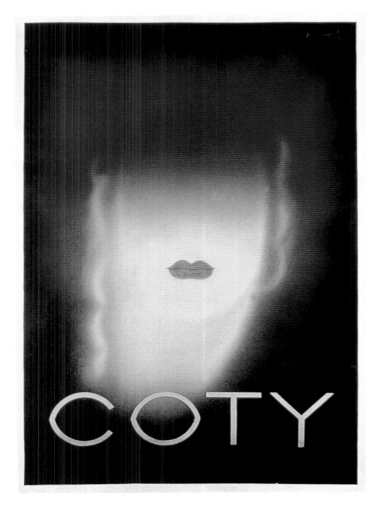

During the first half of this century, many perfume companies hired highly talented artists to create indelible images for their products. Coty was no exception. Artist Charles Loupot painted the haunting image in this 1938 advertisement.

Courtesy of Coty Inc.

professional name from the title of a novel.) As a young man, Coty gravitated to Paris, where he became secretary to a political figure. On his way to and from the office, he struck up an acquaintance with a pharmacist who enjoyed blending fragrances. This exposure was enough to captivate the young Corsican. He made a pilgrimage to Grasse and became affiliated with the firm of Antoine Chiris, where he learned the nuances of each of the flowers and the herbs that the firm used. In time, Coty cultivated a highly developed sense of smell and was soon able to identify every element in a compound.

Coty's working methods have become part of perfume lore. One tale about him concerns a perfume that he produced in 1905, La Rose Jacqueminot, which had the lovely scent of a popular rose hybrid. According to the legend, Coty was piqued by his lack of success in introducing the new product. One day, while attempting to sell it in the department store Le Louvre, he flicked a bottle of the perfume onto the tile floor. The bottle of course broke, the scent was released, and soon everyone wanted to know what that scent was: Coty's career was launched.

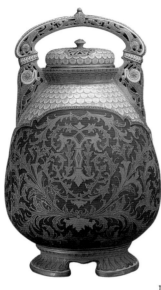

The American firm Ott and Brewer produced this porcelain Belle Époque potpourri jar. Standing 13¹/₂ inches (34.3 cm) tall, it is decorated in polychrome and gold to resemble cloisonné.

Purchase, Barrie A. and Deedee Wigmore Foundation Gift, 1994   1994.46 A-B

By 1910 Coty was considered the most chic perfumer in Paris; his clients included the czar and czarina of Russia, who commissioned fragrances for each of their daughters. Coty's success owed as much to his marketing skills as to his olfactory sense. He was among the first perfumers to give away free samples and to include small bottles in his line, to make his perfumes affordable to young working women. Coty also recognized the importance of the American market and actively cultivated it, at a time when most French firms were nonchalant in their approach. Some of his many successes included Chypre (1907); L'Origan (1907), named for wild marjoram; Jasmin de Corse (1911), named for his birthplace; the oriental-style Emeraude (1923); and L'Aimant, "the magnet" (1927).

PERFUME IN THE TWENTIES

The trend that Poiret started before World War I rapidly expanded during the twenties. Suddenly every major

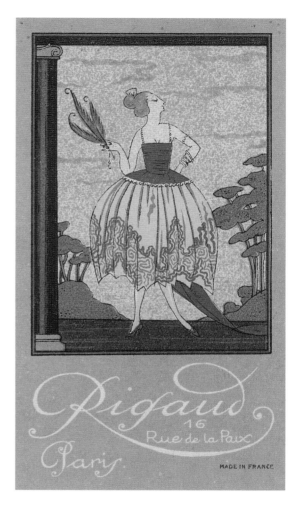

In the early decades of the 20th century, many small perfume companies opened boutiques along the fashionable streets of Paris. This card from Rigaud probably dates to the 1920s.

The Jefferson R. Burdick Collection, Gift of Jefferson R. Burdick   Album 34

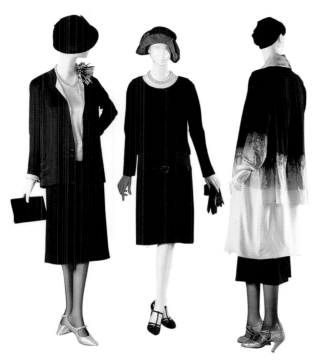

couturier had to have a signature fragrance. This meant substantial growth for the perfume industry in Grasse. Among the most important Parisian designers to join the trend was Gabrielle "Coco" Chanel (1883–1971), whose foray into perfumery became legendary.

Chanel's aesthetic could not have been more opposed to Poiret's exotic ideal. She preferred subdued colors, designs divested of superfluity, and the well-bred look of the British aristocracy. It was her genius to transpose the Englishman's traditional boater hat, tweeds, and patterned Fair Isle pullover into

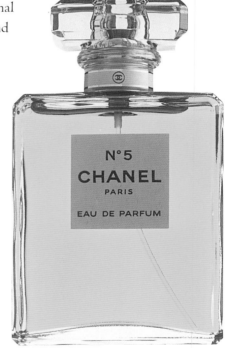

Chanel's soft and beautifully cut garments in wool jersey and silk have become standards, yet each was an innovation in the 1920s. The designs above, from 1926 and 1927, include a day ensemble in black and ivory silk charmeuse, a black wool jersey and black satin day dress, and a theater coat in white and black ombré silk.

Left: Purchase, Gift of the New-York Historical Society, by exchange, 1983 1984.29 A-C
Center: Purchase, Gift of the New-York Historical Society, by exchange, 1983 1984.28 A-C
Right: Purchase, Irene Lewisohn Bequest and Catherine Breyer Von Bomel Foundation, Hoechst Fiber Industries and Chauncey Stillman Gifts, 1984 1984.30
Photograph by Schecter Lee

Most perfume bottles of the 1910s and 1920s featured romantic or floral themes, and so the sleek bottle design for Chanel No. 5 was a sensation when it first appeared. It has barely been altered since. The perfume today, right, has remained among the top sellers since 1921.

Courtesy of Chanel Inc.

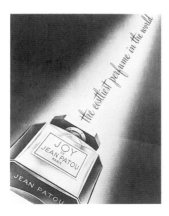

Couturier Jean Patou's Joy was another early triumph in the merging of fashion house and scent. Patou advertised his elegant product as "the costliest perfume in the world," which indeed it was. It is also one of the richest in long-lasting scent.
Courtesy of Jean Patou Inc.

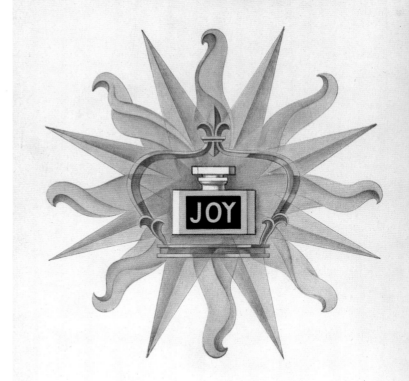

LE PARFUM ROÏ

JEAN PATOU

From the time it was launched in 1931, Joy has been associated with opulence. Here it is advertised as the king of perfumes.
From *Femina*, December 1951. The Metropolitan Museum of Art, The Irene Lewisohn Costume Reference Library

French feminine chic. Chanel and other designers of the twenties created the first tomboy look, which minimized the female form.

Chanel created a major change in perfumery when she collaborated with Ernest Beaux, an emigré from Russia who had worked with the perfume house of Rallet in Moscow, prior to the Russian Revolution in 1917. The two met on the beach at Cannes. Chanel asked Beaux to create a scent for her. He made several, and as the legend goes, she selected the fifth—her lucky number. No. 5 turned out to be an epochal fragrance: Its secret lay in Beaux's addition of small amounts of aldehydes—new, synthetic scents with a brisk ringing note. Beaux also softened and bolstered the blend with a sensitive use of costly naturals, including

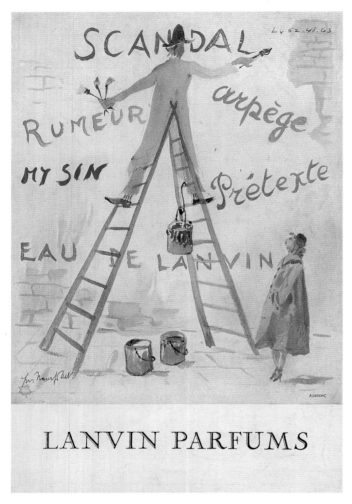

LANVIN PARFUMS

As shown by this ingenious advertisement, the names of Lanvin's perfumes were some of the world's most famous—and infamous.

From *Femina*, October 1951. The Metropolitan Museum of Art, The Irene Lewisohn Costume Reference Library

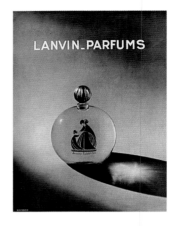

The golden label on this Lanvin perfume bottle depicts Jeanne Lanvin and her daughter dressed for a ball. Before launching into couture, Lanvin designed clothing for children.

Courtesy of Patrimoine Lanvin

ylang-ylang, jasmine, and rose notes. But fine scent was not all there was to the perfume's appeal. Sold in a bottle modeled after one used for a men's cologne, No. 5's look created shock waves, too.

PATOU AND LANVIN

Sportswear was a lucrative line for Chanel as well as for Jean Patou, whose couturier house in Paris further developed the new "spare" look. Patou's original perfume was Amour-Amour, one of the great successes of 1925. Two years later he created the first suntan lotion, Huile de Chaldée (Chaldean Oil), capitalizing on the vogue for sunbathing. (This pastime had been championed by Chanel, who returned to Paris bronzed after a cruise on the duke of Westminster's yacht.)

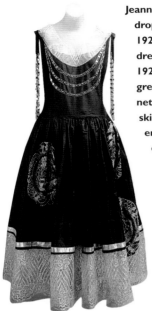

Jeanne Lanvin perfected the dropped-waist style in the 1920s, creating this evening dress in the summer of 1925. It is made of black and green silk with silver-corded net edging on the skirt. The skirt's medallions are embroidered in silk and decorated with paillettes, beads, and faux gems, in imitation of elaborately embroidered Chinese robes.

Gift of Mrs. Albert Spalding, 1962 CI.62.58.1

In 1929 Patou's Le Sien (His) perfume was touted as "a masculine perfume for the outdoors woman," who "plays golf, smokes, and drives a car at 120 [kilometers] an hour." However, the perfume most intimately linked to the name of Patou is Joy, created in 1931. The objective behind the perfume's blending was that it be "free from all vulgarity, cost what it may." And cost it did. Joy made use of the oil of Bulgarian rose and absolute of French jasmine, two of the most expensive ingredients known. It was originally purchased by subscription in limited editions, and advertisements have made much of its distinction as "the world's most expensive perfume."

Sportiness was not the only statement of style in the twenties. The lines of couturier Jeanne Lanvin's dresses and coats were new but not severe. Like Chanel, however, Lanvin enjoyed attracting and working with the top artistic talent of Paris. She had designer Paul Iribe create the famous black bottle for her perfume My Sin—a very racy name at the time of the perfume's launch in 1925. The fragrance was a mixed floral type blended by André Fraysse. In 1927 Fraysse also created Lanvin's famous Arpège, named after a musical arpeggio, which it imitated in its crescendo of olfactory notes. Arpège is a warm, attractive composition, rich in jasmine and other florals.

The success of Shalimar in the early 1920s coincided with a vogue for orientalism. Shalimar's exotic scent set the standard for what an oriental-type perfume should be. The perfume today, right, is one of the most enduringly popular scents.

Courtesy of Guerlain Inc.
Photograph by Jean Baptiste Degez

The house of Guerlain was also extraordinarily active after World War I, particularly in producing oriental-style scents. Mitsouko, a chypre-type perfume with hints of peach, pear, and jasmine, was created during the war and released in 1919. Mitsouko was the name of the tragic Japanese heroine of a popular 1909 romance by French novelist Claude Farrère. In 1925 Guerlain launched the romantic Shalimar, a rich blend of exotic oils, including sandalwood, vetiver, patchouli, civet, and musk. Shalimar also included a modern, synthetic touch of vanilla, for Jacques Guerlain believed that vanilla was an aphrodisiac. The flacon, designed by Raymond Guerlain and made by Baccarat, was modeled after a Mughal garden fountain; the perfume's name was that of the emperor Jahangir's garden in Kashmir.

In 1929, when the house of Guerlain had just passed its centennial anniversary, the company brought out Liù, a floral-bouquet perfume rich in jasmine, ylang-ylang, and of course vanilla. Liù was named after another romantic but tragic heroine, a young Chinese woman who sings a hauntingly beautiful aria before she dies, in Puccini's opera *Turandot*. For all of the brassiness of the Jazz Age—or perhaps because of it—there was still a real market for the romance of make-believe and faraway places.

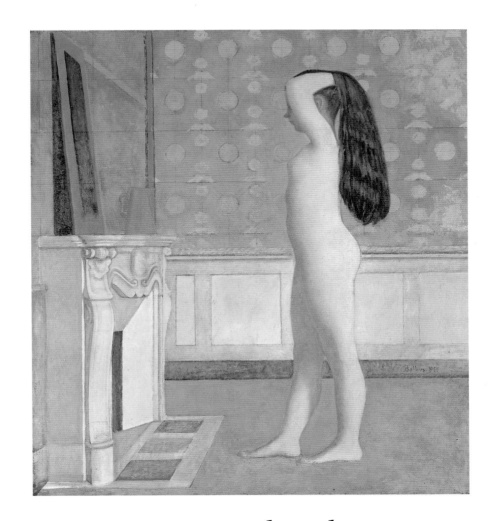

Scent from the Thirties
to the Present

⊱─◈─◆─○─◆─◈─⊰

Scent in the Thirties and Forties

The tomboy look of the twenties gave women an alternative to more traditional styles, but by the thirties, another voice was insisting that "the body must never be forgotten." Italian-born Elsa Schiaparelli, who opened her couture shop in Paris at the end of the twenties, was both aristocrat and rebel. She chose the finest fabrics and draped them beautifully, but as she liked to say, she also enjoyed "setting off firecrackers." A friend of many Surrealist artists, Schiaparelli shared their love of the offbeat. Schiaparelli's mentor was Poiret, and like him, she saw fashion as theater.

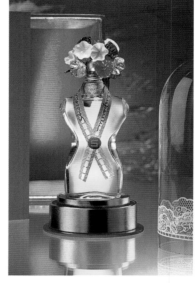

Elsa Schiaparelli achieved her desired effect when she presented Shocking in a bottle shaped like the female form.

Courtesy of Schiaparelli Inc.

Shocking pink was Schiaparelli's favorite color, and Shocking was the name she chose for her 1937 perfume, a fragrance based on patchouli, a scent that was rarely used in the 1930s. Schiaparelli's perfumer, Jean Amic, from the Grasse firm of Roure Bertrand Dupont, was one of the great scent composers of the century. Shocking's bottle design was supposedly based on the film star Mae West's well-known silhouette.

Schiaparelli's 1938 evening cape was inspired by the Neptune Fountain in the Parc de Versailles.

Bequest of Lady Mendl, 1951
CI.51.83

On the previous page is *Figure in Front of a Mantel*, a 1955 painting by Balthus (Count Balthasar Klossowski de Rola).

Robert Lehman Collection, 1975
1975.1.155

The thirties also saw the introduction of several other perfume classics. Tabu, formulated by Jean Carles for the Spanish firm of Dana, was sumptuous and oriental. (Similar fragrance notes are also found in Estée Lauder's Youth Dew and Yves Saint Laurent's Opium.) In 1933, the house of Dana produced Twenty Carats—a perfume in lieu of the diamonds that few could afford during the Depression years. Jacques Guerlain captured the era's fascination with flight by naming his spicy new perfume Vol de Nuit (Night Flight), after the title of a popular book by French aviator Antoine de Saint Exupéry.

PERFUMERY IN THE 1940S

The years of World War II were dark for all French luxury industries. Few new fragrances were created, because perfumers were cut off from the aromatics they needed in India and the East Indies and from markets in America and Britain. Nevertheless, Houbigant's Chantilly (1941), Raphael's Réplique (1944), and Mademoiselle Cellier's innovative Bandit (1944) appeared. In 1944, Edmond Roudnitska, who was soon to become the perfumer to Dior, also produced Femme for the house of Rochas, and in 1945 Jacqueline Fraysse created Antilope for the house of Weil.

Before the Great Depression and World War II, couture and its ancillary arts like perfume were France's second highest export. At the end of the war, the French government intervened in the fashion business to help recover financial losses, financing in 1945 a show called Théâtre de la Mode. Sent throughout the world, the show was built around miniature mannequins and elaborate painted sets that displayed France's greatest resource, the work of its finest designers.

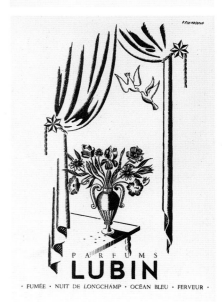

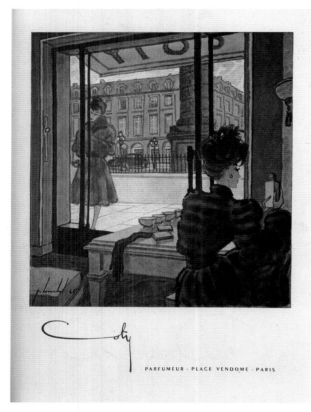

This advertisement shows Coty's shop in Paris as it looked in the 1940s.

From *La Femme Chic*, December 1945. The Metropolitan Museum of Art, Irene Lewisohn Costume Reference Library

Among these designers were formidable talents such as Pierre Balmain, Cristóbal Balenciaga, Marcel Rochas, and Nina Ricci, all of whom would launch great perfumes.

DIOR AND THE POSTWAR REVIVAL

As part of the postwar revival effort, the French textile firm of Boussac gave extensive financing to Christian Dior. In what seemed a single stroke, Dior abolished the efficient, trim clothing of the war years, replacing it with the New Look, which he launched on February 12, 1947. Sweeping skirts, tiny waists, and bare shoulders returned in full splendor, as though the empress Eugénie had taken to the runway in her crinolines and décolleté.

Dior's work was meticulous, calling for both new couture techniques and the rediscovery of others that had not been used since the turn of the century. The world was tired of the Depression and war, so the New Look was a coup for France.

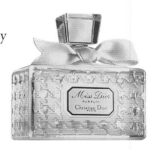

Miss Dior, above, followed upon the triumphant success of Dior's New Look, appearing in 1947 as the couturier's first perfume.

Courtesy of Christian Dior Perfumes

Parisian couturiers took orders for new styles, while the fashion industry elsewhere resisted or tried to catch up. The perfume industry, of course, rode on fashion's coattails. Dior introduced Miss Dior perfume in 1947. It was the first of many illustrious Dior scents to be created by Edmond

Roudnitska at his laboratory at Cabris. The fragrance Diorama made its appearance in 1949 and Diorissimo in 1955.

Among the other great perfumes of the period was Cristóbal Balenciaga's rich, floral Le Dix, which debuted in 1947. In 1948 Robert Ricci designed the famous twin doves for Nina Ricci's spicy, floral L'Air du Temps. In the next decade, Audrey Hepburn inspired Givenchy's 1957 L'Interdit, and the house of Balmain produced Miss Balmain in 1958. The following year, couturier Madame Grès asked her perfumer, Omar Arif, to create a fragrance that would evoke her trip through the Spice Islands. The result was Cabochard, an exotic blend that has become a classic.

Dior's fashions, like this 1949 Junon gown, restored the glamour of the Belle Époque.
Gift of Mrs. Byron C. Foy, 1953
CI 53.40.5 A-E

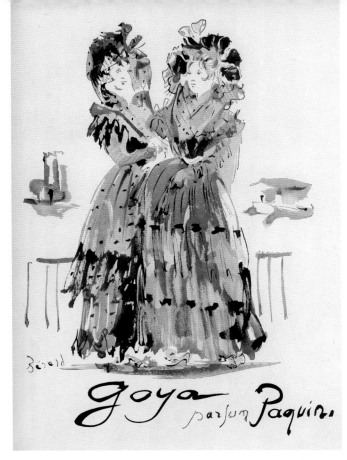

The advertisement above is for a perfume by Paquin, one of many Parisian fashion houses that produced fine fragrances.
From *La Femme Chic*, December 1946. The Metropolitan Museum of Art, Irene Lewisohn Costume Reference Library

In New York, Estée Lauder's perfumery career was launched in 1953 with Youth Dew. Her marketing was very clever. Knowing that American women did not like to spend money on luxuries like perfume but did like the pleasures of the bath, Lauder did not try to sell them a perfume at all. Youth Dew was produced as a bath oil

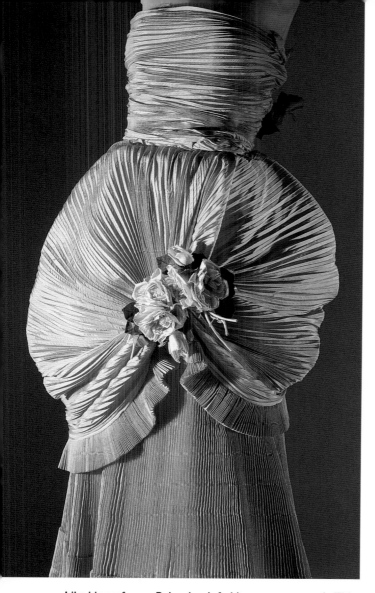

Like his perfumes, Balenciaga's fashions were romantic. This gown, shown in detail, was from his winter 1947 collection.

Gift of Lisa and Jody Greene, in memory of their loving mother, Ethel S. Greene, 1958   CI.58.13.6 A-B

and was readily accepted. Richly scented with an oriental blend of frankincense, patchouli, vetiver, clove, and musk, it is one of the three best-selling perfumery products of all time in America.

THE SIXTIES AND BEYOND

The 1960s were an unsettling though exciting decade for the luxury industries. The great master Christian Dior had died in 1957, and his young successor, Yves Saint Laurent, embraced the new informality in fashion. Other designers followed with ready-to-wear lines. Perfumes that reflected the uninhibited mood of the times included Guy Laroche's Fidji in 1966 and Paco Rabanne's Calandre in 1969. The decade's youth rebellion and the subsequent women's movement helped to create changes in the way that perfumes were marketed. In 1973 Charles Revson had a tremendous success with the launch of Charlie, a perfume whose ads featured—for the first time—an independent young woman wearing pants. As the decade progressed, France ceased to be the sole center for perfumery; the United States emerged as a major fragrance trendsetter and producer.

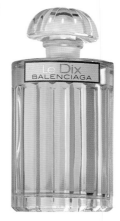

Balenciaga's romantic and floral Le Dix, above, debuted in 1947.

Courtesy of Balenciaga Inc.

What began with Poiret and Chanel in Paris—the couturier as perfumer—finally caught on in New York in the 1970s. Every major designer of the day—Geoffrey Beene, Halston, Oscar de la Renta, Diane von Furstenberg—brought out a perfume as the olfactory essence of their style. Designer perfumes today account for more than forty percent of perfume sales. In the 1980s and 1990s, Italian, British, and Japanese designers joined their French and American counterparts in producing signature fragrances. At the same time, new areas emerged as major perfume consumers, notably Spain, Brazil, Mexico, Eastern Europe, and above all, the Pacific Rim countries.

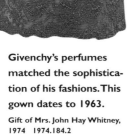

Givenchy's perfumes matched the sophistication of his fashions. This gown dates to 1963.
Gift of Mrs. John Hay Whitney, 1974 1974.184.2

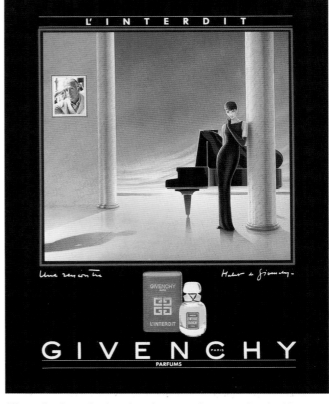

L'Interdit, shown in the advertisement above, was inspired by Audrey Hepburn in 1957 and is still associated with her image.
Courtesy of Parfums Givenchy

RECENT TRENDS

With the vast interest in fitness and health in the late twentieth century, there have been many new directions in perfumery. The trends have been toward sharp, clear, "ozonic" scents, as well as outdoorsy or "oceanic" scents. In general these perfumes have a more unisex appeal than those of the past. In 1992 Dior introduced Dune, with notes of the sea reinforced with florals. Calvin Klein's Escape is another "clean" perfume, although it contains hyacinth, citrus, and fruit notes as well. At the same time, traditional floral, oriental, green, and chypre-type perfume favorites still challenge all newcomers.

Perfume companies gather new botanical products in the South American rainforest, in Malaysia, South Africa, Indonesia, China, and other sites, and they develop new technologies as well. Headspace, a chromatographic process perfected in the 1970s, enables scientists in a laboratory to analyze a living plant and identify the molecules responsible for its scent. With even more recent computer technology, the scent of a plant can be analyzed in its natural setting. This immediacy allows perfumers to re-create a scent more closely than ever before.

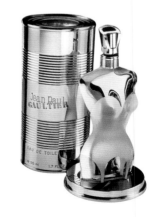

Jean Paul Gaultier brought exoticism into the 1990s through his perfume and clothing designs. He created these Tartar coat-and-pant ensembles in 1994 using vibrant silks and satins, fur and fake fur.
Gifts of Richard Martin, 1995
LEFT: 1995.433.9 A-C
RIGHT: 1995.433.10 A-B

In France, the real-estate boom in the Riviera has spelled the end of many of the great plantations of jasmine and tuberose, but elsewhere fields devoted to roses, jasmine, and other perfumery plants have expanded tremendously. India and China grow many new fragrance crops, as do Tasmania and North Africa.

The bottle still reigns. In marketing the perfume V'E, Versace produced a limited-edition Baccarat crystal flacon, left.
Courtesy of Versace Profumi Ltd.

Jean Paul Gaultier's torso bottle and "tin can" container, right, were meant to shock, like the designer's fashions.
Courtesy of Boucheron Ltd.

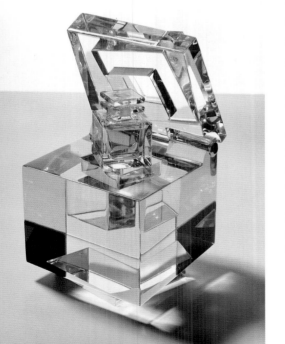

THE BEAUTY OF THE BOTTLE

Issey Miyake's bottles for L'Eau d'Issey, above, exemplify the minimalist trends of modern perfumery packaging.
Courtesy of Boucheron Ltd.

As the perfume industry and scent preferences have diversified in the twentieth century, the importance of creating beautiful bottles to hold scented products has remained constant. Almost every new bottle reflects thought, imagination, and fineness of materials. Standouts have included bottles that are unusual (Jaipur, Jean Paul Gaultier), minimalist (L'Eau d'Issey, Obsession), sculptural (Niki de St. Phalle, Deci Delà), lacquerlike (Armani, Opium), or decorated with gold (Polo, Zen). Packaging is a significant factor in the price of a perfume and is often more costly than its essential oils. Within the industry, certain names are synonymous with great artistry in package creation. In Paris, Serge Mansau was responsible for Vivre, Septième Sens, and Infini, among others. Pierre Dinand bottle designs include those for Ivoire, Coriandre, and Kouros. Although René Lalique died shortly after World War II, his atelier continues to produce beautiful flacons, as does the house of Baccarat.

Today the major implementers of fragrance-bottle design are located in France. Yet as always—just as in the days of Cleopatra, Caterina de' Medici, and Madame de Pompadour—independent artists and glassblowers throughout the world are creating one-of-a-kind containers to hold scents that are also one of a kind.

Artists continue to design perfume bottles as unique pieces of sculpture. *Kinesthesis Bottle*, right, was made by the American artist William Carlson in 1981.
Gift of Douglas and Michael Heller, in memory of Eleanor Heller, 1981   1981.234

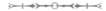

We would like to thank the following people:

Geoffrey R. Webster, Cosimo Policastro, Lisa Popoli,
Lori Smith, Cheryle Puso, and the perfumers of Givaudan Roure
Fragrances for their generosity and expertise in creating the
eight historical fragrances for *Scents of Time*;

Donatella Giacometti, Liza Ross Dousson, and Stacy Haymes
at KCSA Worldwide for their help and enthusiasm;

Georges Gotlib of Gotlib Design and Resources
for his advice and guidance;

Annette Green of The Fragrance Foundation for her support.

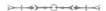